FROM THE ROOTS

FROM THE ROOTS

The True Story of How I Beat Death
and Learned to Live

MARSHA THERESE DANZIG

Skyhorse Publishing

Skyhorse Publishing books may be purchased in bulk at special discounts for sales promotion, corporate gifts, fund-raising, or educational purposes. Special editions can also be created to specifications. For details, contact the Special Sales Department, Skyhorse Publishing, 307 West 36th Street, 11th Floor, New York, NY 10018 or info@skyhorsepublishing.com.

Visit our website at www.skyhorsepublishing.com.

10 9 8 7 6 5 4 3 2 1

Library of Congress Cataloging-in-Publication Data is available on file.

Cover design by Jane Sheppard
Cover photo: iStockphoto

Print ISBN: 978-1-5107-1291-1
Ebook ISBN: 978-1-5107-1295-9

Printed in the United States

Dedicated to Faith, Hope, and Love

CONTENTS

Chapter 1

Speak. Speak. Speak. You tell your story.
You get that suffering spoken for.
You get that hope out there.

You tell the world how you have won, over and over, and have not succumbed.
This is worthwhile, says He. I trust Him, for once.
Open. Open Open.

Open.

Open.

Open.

Open.

Open.

Open.

The diagnosis is not good, so they say. I am five. It is the sixties. So much death anxiety is associated with that word: cancer. I'd never heard of it before. As the adults swarm around me, day in, day out, kiddie-gloving their way around the little girl (or muscle), mounting my will, I vaguely sense that I am very seriously . . . not well.

A life-size clown doll is propped up in the hospital bed next to beaming, smiling me. The two of us sit. Our smiles are real. What do I know?

I know cancer only has meaning because someone gave it meaning. And so it goes, my lifetime of overwhelm, tension, and extreme holding to stay away from, divert attention from, please God keep me from, cancer. I still don't know what it really means.

I receive bedloads of presents for something I must have done.
Oh, I know! I have cancer!

How did I get from hospital beds to this moment? I have some idea . . . but I leave that up to God to tell me someday.

Accept This.

A pearl dropped from heaven

The earth opened up and swallowed her whole

And when she'd had her fill of sustaining and nurturing

She loosened her grip

The pearl walked the earth

Each bare footstep

Echoed

"Don't forget. Don't forget. Don't ever forget!"

CHAPTER 2

There is no separation from the love of God.

"I will prune you, cultivate you, water you. This will be hard. Behold you are gold in the palm of my hand."

Belief always starts in the body.

Before Christmas, I found the presents. I sat among them, wrapping paper piled high above my tiny head. I kept a few of the dolls, even though I knew they were for my sister. I cut their hair. Pure delight.

Children didn't come over much after the diagnosis. I continued to have a habit of playing beauty shop. Little girls with long, bright blond curls would be dropped off. Mothers came to pick them up; the same little girls bounding to the door, excited about their new hairdo. I wanted them to look like me.

When I returned to school in the middle of first grade, a girl lost her contact lens. I did not know what a contact lens was. I only knew it was slightly invisible. How would they find the invisible? She had a problem, like me, only I was all better. The teacher treated me delicately. I was separate. And special.

I met love in the mirror
I stepped forward just 10, then 20, then 3,000 feet
I touched my hand to the flame and I was not burned

This is Gratitude
To look into the mirror
See Death
And reflect back resurrection

This is knowledge
To look in the mirror
And see only Christ

This is suffering
To turn your back
From the mirror

CHAPTER 3

Life is too short

Dress Up

Eleanor had very nice clothing, so one day I walked to her apartment. The door was open, but no one was inside. I grabbed as many items as my five-year-old body could drag down the stairs and *ran* back to my house. For hours I stood in my backyard trying on her clothes, pretending to be her. I hid the pile from my mother, who brought me orange slices. I wore the orange slices like lipstick, the juice oozing down Eleanor's exquisite dresses and tiny white lace blouses. Her parents came to collect the goods eventually. I never felt bad about what I had done. I had a right to look pretty, too.

Eleanor moved out of her apartment. A blond hippie moved in. I started going to her house to learn songs by Mary Hopkin and Joni Mitchell. She gave me an Apple 45 rpm record. My dachshund chewed it, but I played it anyway. No one knew I went to the hippie's apartment after school. I was in second grade. The whole school was looking for me. My mother was looking for me. I moseyed on home around four on a Thursday afternoon. I had my own life to lead.

Heave

Go by inner flow

Whisper medicine of

Love, Rhythm, Soul

Beneath a laugh full of remedy

Look through winter dream

Night mind

Use your beauty

Black cocktail gown

Truth bed

Bella red

CHAPTER 4

This childhood is blurry. I don't remember much.
Who my first grade teacher was,
what my classmates' names were, what I learned in kindergarten.
I remember . . .
The blades of grass.

This one sat in the front seat of the station wagon on Cambridge Road.
Somehow the car was turned on, but the blade could not steer.
This blade swung on the backyard swings
when Father Joe met her for the first time.
Now she knew what truly handsome was.
This blade sipped iced coffee from her father's cup.

This blade did a lot of ungodly manner-free
activities that embarrassed numerous adults.
This blade rode on the back of her calico cat, Holly.

This blade turned the pink plastic crown
of the dancing doll. Hoping against hope.
This blade touched the sticky pine trees near her house.

This blade sat complacent, coloring, on her grandmother's front porch.

Rims of sadness surround pain and fear.
Worry, seeded in large clumps, moves
in its own direction, away from the flow.

It is hard work to find the blades of joy, laughter, hilarity,
lightness, peace, contentment, happiness, love. But I always do.

I have often coated each sorry blade with the cloak of fierce hope.
So I could own my own happiness after every broken moment.

I step back.

If He can walk through it with wide open heart,
perhaps there are others who can enjoy the beauty won by arduous grace.

I see the wind blowing the weight
of a remembered life in metaphors and sensations.
The wind blows where it will.
The field continues to grow. I love this life.

After I slipped off the balance beam during gym, I did not want to go to the school doctor, but they made me. This was more than a sprain, with swelling, heat, the familiar hard protuberance cluttering my left ankle. I already knew it was back.

My mother was on the phone with someone important. She kept mentioning my name.

I went into the piano room. I was searching for the keys to play. Bach, Mozart, a Turkish Rondo, and "Free Man in Paris."

Something to know. To make me feel.

I couldn't play.

I stared at the white grand piano as the sun kept its guard.

There was a meeting of two types of light, and I was caught in the crossfire, the gray area.

She called me back into the kitchen. I already knew what was coming, but I had to hear her words.

Boston . . . Children's Hospital . . . biopsy . . . right away . . . can't wait. Nothing about tumor. Nothing about C.

Cancer is the word, the scar, the great wondering. I bring cancer along with me, in one shape or another, to every potential friend.

I don't know how to do friendship. I am missing some skills.

I want friends so I give them a try in a worried, hyper sort of way.

Will I be too clingy? Will I cry too much or not enough? This is a girl who just three years earlier had been strapped to a crib, a net covering her so she wouldn't escape. Oh, the embarrassment of it!

The day after Christmas my father took us to the Jersey Shore. The other kids were complaining about the cold and wind. I wanted to stay all day, not get in that car again. Would this be the last time I had fresh air?

Life loved her right back, and her doubts diminished. Life loved her right back, and she was watched over in the rain.

Life loved her right back, and she found she had skin that glistened.

Life loved her right back, and she was never alone.
Life loved her right back, and she could sit in silence safely.

Life loved her right back, and her territory expanded.
Life loved her right back, and her tenderness was a strength.

Life loved her right back, and she was welcomed in unfamiliar places.

Life loved her right back, and she belonged.

Chapter 5

When do I get to have a girlfriend who helps me with my hair,
makeup, and clothing, who does fundraisers to help me during chemo,
who is jealous of ME sometimes and tells me because we're just that cool?

When do I get to walk into a room with a posse, rather than alone?

When do I get to have help when I feel tremendously awkward?

When do I get to shine in all my glory
without worrying I will lose friends?

When do I get to be noticed?

When do I get to have a boyfriend?

When do I get to feel pretty?

When do I get to have a great social life with lots of friends
who can't wait to see me?

When do I get to be in Seventeen *magazine?*
When do I get to be welcomed?

When do I get to look good in all my outfits
and turn boys' heads wherever I go?

When do I get to tell everyone that the most popular
girl in school is actually really mean and manipulative
and how come nobody can see that?

When do I get to tell someone, straight to their face, that they are so full of shit it isn't even funny?

We moved to a small suburb of Albany, New York. I walked to school in the morning. After school I went wherever I wanted to go, usually walking the borders of the road as if I were walking a balance beam. Angie, my new friend, had a Ouija board. Her maid from Trinidad practiced voodoo. Angie smoked cigarettes in third grade. We did a lot of nasty things.

White go-go boots are worn. Astrakhan, embroidered, woven winter coats are plopped on my medium-size body. I learn how to knit. I bake tiny cakes in my Easy-Bake Oven. My favorite song is anything that is not popular. I love anything in a minor key. No one else does.

I did a lot of bad things: stole batteries from Radio Shack, bit my friend Hope, played doctor with various boys in the neighborhood, locked my terrified sister Darcy in a tree house, threw things at a kid who has Tourette's, lit illegal fireworks, stole pornography and looked at it with my friends, tore apart someone's tent with a knife, lied about how long I practiced piano. At least I didn't try to drown anyone like Angie did me.

Angie and I had a séance in my father's closet, calling back the recent spirit of my dead grandfather, Joseph Michael. I never liked him much. He was so angry, but he was the only dead person I knew. My father had a bag of PG cigar wraps in a bag in his closet. If he got enough wraps, he got prizes. Above the bag were all his laundered shirts.

We called out to the spirit of Joseph, "If you are here, make your presence known." The shirts began to move. We were both oddly excited. We were so powerful.

Encouraged, we went outside to try our hand at the weather. We marched in a circle, chanting what we supposed were "Indian" songs. Our neighbor came by.

"What are you girls up to?"

"We are calling on the spirit of rain to come down." It began to rain a few minutes later.

Our neighbor came out again in the rain.

"Why don't you do a dance to make the sun come out?"

So we did. The sun came out. Assured of our great power to tame nature, we went upstairs to dress the Infant of Prague in pretty, silk-collared robes, thanking the baby Jesus for all his goodness.

Feel the wind in long branches

Succumb to rain and storm

Trust in good news

Sapling wings

Ancestor worship

Allow unbending

Full

Guided

Withstanding

Give

Unending

Before I knew any different, I was happy to be happy.

I ran.

I jumped.

I laughed.

I hid only for play.

I liked the attention my smiles produced.

I was silly at inopportune moments.

I trusted . . . my father, my mother, little girls, little boys, dogs, cats, rodents.

I was the tree, the fruit, the branches, the roots,
the bark, the stems, the berries, the thorns, the seeds.

I was the tree missing twigs and buds.

I was the tree among others.

I did not tell myself:

You are not enough to exist as is.

You have too many scars to be beautiful.

You are unwelcome in these parts.

You are too inexperienced for your aged branches.

You don't know what to do.

You won't be helped.

You are not as pretty as that tree, or that one, or that one.

Your success is measured by the number of leaves you possess.

You can be torn down easily; this world is so unfriendly.

You are too sensitive to the elements.

You aren't well-bred.

You don't hold your branches correctly.

You have no faith.

You have not produced enough seeds.

You are too accepting of your circumstances.

You are allowing others to encroach upon your space. Protect!

You are not following your divine purpose.

You are too serious. It is just a branch. Get over it.

You are responsible for the ones who planted you.

You must be vigilant.

You are not allowed to rest when there is so much work to be done.

You should not be too grand.

You have no right to enjoy the sun when others are hurting.

You need to be stronger.

In those former days,

I was naked and unashamed.

I knelt before the Sacred Oak.

I loved her.

I was naked still.

So was she.

CHAPTER 6

The bird's wing was caught in the pavement
Her wings flapped uncontrollably, her eyes staring off
Her talons, hooked into the small granules of molten tar, trapped her
She was in the center of the storm,
That place where anyone could trample her dreams
Or end her life
As I reached down to release her talons and wing out of the tar,
She surrendered
Her airy frame and downy soft body surprised me
I expected her to be heavier
I took her to a rock at the edge of the road
She staggered for a moment, shook out her wings, and took off,
her back toward me
Sometimes freedom needs our help to fly.

I never feel like I am drowning when I swim. My butterfly stroke is powerful. My shoulders are huge. As I get older, that is somehow not an asset for a girl. Who knew? I compete with myself, under the water, to the edge of the pool. I am everything I cannot completely be above water—free flowing, fiercely strong, vocal, determined, pushy, alone without it being some conditional fault of mine.

Someone in fifth grade stains a desk with her blood. I hope the teacher doesn't make me sit there. Other than that, I just don't care. I don't care what I wear, how I act, who likes me. I have my bad girl posse. I wear no socks in February.

There were very few days when I was not upside down, all those years on 7 Imperial Drive. I started with handstand holds against the wall. They evolved into hand-walking marathons down the curved driveway in front of our slate-gray suburban home. First fifty steps, one hundred, then two hundred. Handstands led to backflips, front flips, handsprings, back handsprings.

I practiced back- and front flips until I got them. I was constantly spraining a finger or an ankle. I didn't care. I twirled everywhere. I could run a front flip over my family room couch, landing on the hardwood floor. Backflips off the diving board were a piece of cake. Butterfly was my favorite stroke. My bell-bottoms were torn into rags at the bottom, dragged with mud. The other girls were discovering makeup. I didn't understand. Who cared about what a boy thought of you when you could do a full aerial into a backflip then top it off with a handspring? Could any of the boys in my eighth grade class do that?

My parents went out for a late dinner. My older sister, a teenager, decided to have a party. There was kissing and drinking and loud music. She told me to go upstairs, leave her alone, and especially not to tell Mom and Dad. I went outside to our flat backyard, where I began to walk on my hands back and forth, underneath the wide window in the "party room." All the kids could see were my feet, going back and forth. My sister was not happy, but I kept it up, using blackmail:"If you make me stop, I will tell."

I wouldn't have noticed the rocky lump in my ankle if it had not been for backflips.

I would not have noticed the flaming red of my lower left bones or the swollen mass of flesh that I could penetrate with deep thumbprints, if it had not been for the handsprings. I would not have done anything if it weren't for the day my father noticed that lump, the one he had seen on that same ankle in 1967. I said it was nothing, but I already knew. Anything to hold on. Anything.

If I open

Will I be remembered?

If I try nothing
But stand
Fingers spread
Saying, "Hear me. Let me be seen."

Will I be a fortress still?
Where is that root of strength encouraging me

Power
Free
I can only wait one more second
The breath has ended
Another is on its way

Now. Fear. Now. Don't stop. Now. Leaf unfolding. Now.

Ready.

Chapter 7

Needs More Filling

I stopped in the road

The same question

Running, running, running

I want to turn away from it

It never goes away

Sometimes I turn my back

To try to face my God

Turn my back from the question

And be a good girl

Positive, hopeful, alive

But how can I continue my road

If I don't overcome the question

It doesn't matter really

God is everywhere I go

God and the question

I have made my decision

The void of negativity

My supposed hopelessness and desperate frustration

Is a waiting vessel

Womb of the deepest type ever

Every depressed belief is a prayer waiting

It is the ultimate hope, my repetitive question

With an opportunity to receive the grandest filling

I long to fill you up, says God

Goodness for the weary wounds

Hope, Hope, Hope

Hope is in the question

Hope will set me free

I was in love with:

- Patrick McGoohan—*The Prisoner*. He was trapped on an island. He did not know who was for him or against him. He wore slick black suits. He drove an Aston Martin. He smirked often and made flourishing movements. Someday I would live in Europe and fall in love with a swashbuckler.
- Tolstoy—He was so self-righteous and angry.
- Molière—He had a good BS meter.
- Saint-Exupéry—He dreamed big.

I have to find a way to swallow small as I am led into the bright chemo room with all the other kids waiting to be served. I will never accept this. Chemo hurts every time.

I was beginning to make my own necessary split between two lives: one that would be medical, and one that would try with all possible strength to be everything else. It didn't take the doctors too long to form a diagnosis. The cancer seemed to jump from the petri dish screaming, "See me, see me."

A lot of silence wheeled me into the small room. The surgeon used words. I know he did. All I saw was the side of his hand, landing formidably at the upper portion of my left shin. My left leg recoiled.

I know that night came. There was a waking up. And a father sitting to my right. A much smaller, younger child emerged.

"Why Daddy, why?" I have never seen my father sob since then.

My clinking, metal cane with the black rubber tip had holes in it to line up with my height.

The physical therapists wanted me to get off the crutches, but I was so good at using them! Swinging between steps, plopping onto my bottom to sit. Was I ready? Was I ready?!

They insisted at the Institute that I needed to evolve from the crutches, that crutches would hold me back, that I COULD walk again.

All that summer I tried my best. By the time I was brought back to school in December, after six months of intensive chemotherapy, I decided I needed to look like I was not limping too much. I didn't want the girls to ask a lot of questions.

I used the cane like a baton when I wasn't leaning on it. I could count the knobs on the metal frame, sticking my finger pads in just enough to feel the defined edges of the metal. I should have been done with the cane by the end of sophomore year, but I insisted on using it until senior year, when my hair finally came back. Anything to hold on to. Anything.

Today I stood on solid ground, without shoes, without socks.

Just molecules of flesh touching reconnected flesh billions of years old.

I tried to reach the lava pit, but something was missing
from the external fire that broiled from below.

It was the part of me, cut off, disconnected, that stopped
at the line where I was supposed to get to harmony.

I was off-center.

What was on the left, what remained, was man-made.

The decaying flesh that would serve for grass one
million years from now had been emptied of life,

Formaldehyde-treated, preserved in its disease.

I wondered, when it transformed itself, in the centuries
to come, would the curse still be there always blocking
one eternal soul from the core of the earth?

Perhaps I must look upward

Perhaps the ground on which I stand cannot
decay but you cannot see it.

I ask you, Jesus Christ, what did they do with
my leg the day my life became a form of loss?

When will I see it again?

How will it manifest itself within my body, its replacement?

It has always been there, but I cannot see it any longer.

Jesus died. He rose three days later, whole.

I am resurrected in the new life, too, where an appendage is frivolous.

Perhaps someday I will have ten or twenty legs on which to dance.

And the thread that I always thought was missing,

as I could not feel the earth beneath my arched foot,

is now the song I knew when I was just a thought.

CHAPTER 8

I am the coiled life that lifts the angel's wings
and the devil of your darkest desires down below
I swirl through sea creatures, dance in swinging limbs

I drown you in my hidden knowledge,
and then float you to the surface, unscathed
I can crawl upon the ground unnoticed,
then strike you where it hurts the most,
only to stir you, only to make you sweat again.

Sweet sweet sweat of life
I am merciless pleasure
Sympathy and soul
Seething with craving
I strangle you whole, to protect you from your own illusions

I separate you from all that is not sacred
I wrap myself around your fears and show you the way out
Through long-necked giraffes, well-rooted trees, swirls of paint on a page,
a reed blowing in the wind,
a jaguar tail wrapped around a Kapok branch, a number in a lineup,
a peacock feather

I find you
I am both beginning and end.
This is hard.
I am every act of integrity ever witnessed.
I am the whip on his precious back, and the spine
that lets him carry the weight
Nations rise and fall because of me, but they have not known me.
I mean no harm. I am the nectar of life itself. Wake me up. You will see.

I am she. I am she. I am SHE.

College. After three semesters I am bleeding internally. And why wouldn't I be?

I have fallen in love with Jesus. I drown in Christian conservative theology. I am a walking referee for God. What to do with all the lesbians on campus? And women who do not believe in God? Horror!

One day I am bent over at the back of my kidneys, unable to cross the lawn from my car to class. I shouldn't be standing at all. I just have to get back to the car after class. I tell no one about the hourly trips to the toilet to hemorrhage my little life away. I am a bit tired. My outfits are really cute. I wear a lot of red. Amy, my roommate, is never around. She is an adult.

College Christians have one another. I treasure one girl who seems free and screwed up at the same time. With a straight face she tells our group how she "witnesses about Jesus" when she is out at bars partying. I just love her, but apparently I am not supposed to. Marianne, and all my Christian friends, are popular and somewhat holy. I mean, who says, "What are your spiritual plans for the year?" They pray for me, but they also gossip a lot about one another, and are very physically fit with nice clothes. They marry well, and conservatively, sons of senators, heads of arms-dealing companies, that sort of thing. I find this slightly confusing. What about my Jewish father? He seems nice enough . . . and transparent.

I think I am not a very good Christian at the time. The weight of not having enough faith to be healed begins to drain my spirit soon after I join up with the damn Protestants.

Before, I just ate Jesus.

I know how to stand when others would have fallen. Ha. I think Jesus sees this. We have a moment.

Good morning light
It is time for your unfolding
You have been asleep for far too long
Covered up by roses and lemons and happy thoughts
Depressed cavities that the other tried to fill with what she thought was you
But you know better
Yes, light, it is time for you to come out
No longer hidden
No longer afraid
By what "they" might say
You have no choice
The day has come
It is no longer night
You have been with her for a very long time
Full of desire
Yet daring not to shine
She is too full of you now
Come out and share your wealth
The world is waiting . . .

CHAPTER 9

Little girl got very lost in the big city. She saw: Tall buildings
Crazy people
Pretty, well-dressed women with handsome men on their arms
Decorated apartments
Icy bus stops

Evening gowns not worn by her
Large signs shouting out glamorous events that
she hoped she'd be invited to
Moneyed pockets
Bay windows
Dust
Sexy electric company workers lining up for hot pretzels and coffee
Statues, so many statues

She took a deep breath, wrapped her cashmere scarf around
her shivering shoulders, and stepped out into the cold.

There was a place in the center of her belly, where
the mother should have been.

I tried to walk up the stairs, to get to French class.

"Always stop at the water fountain on the right, Marsha. Sip at least one cup. That way you won't have to go back."

It wasn't that far, the top of the stairs to the end of the pale pink and gray hall with the seafoam green walls. Thank God I had Madame as my teacher. The other one, that Norwegian, had such a horrible accent.

Madame's room was set up like a French café, only of the Catholic school variety. Stiff metal desks, crosses everywhere, posters of the Champs-Élysées, fields of lavender and a man wearing a beret, riding a bike, baguette popping out of his jacket. At least Madame wasn't a nun.

We were studying the subjunctive. It would be . . . It could be . . . It could change. Pout pout. French. French. Horsey lips breathing and a wave of the hand. Vive la discipline!

I knew I would be fluent. But I also wondered if I could make it back down the stairs.

Class ended. Time for another cup.

Please may no one see me now. I can do this. May they not hear my heavy heaving.

Down the stairs I went.

I stopped at the bench in the front hallway. No one must know.

I can't go back; I can't go back.

That past weekend I had gone to a party at Faith's. Why didn't I remember to flush the toilet? She called my mother.

It was a temporary problem that would get better, this hemorrhaging. I convinced my mother it hadn't happened before, a mere symptom of chemo.

I had been hemorrhaging for months.

It was just a little bit more of a walk to the school library; there was a private bathroom in the back. I could spend some time there, trying to push the blood clots out of my urethra.

Twenty minutes later I was out of the bathroom, cornered. The librarian, my friend Jen, Faith, and the guidance counselor.

"Marsha, you are white as a ghost; you need to get home."

They called and they called my mother. My father was out of town.

No one was answering.

"I'll be all right. Call me a taxi and I'll get home."

I sat in the back of that gassy taxi breathing rapidly.

The taxi driver pulled into the driveway. My mother's car was there. And another car.

I couldn't even make it to the side door.

Let me tell you about the front door.

#1 The doorbell was as faint as my voice.

#2 The door was inches thick.

#3 When a girl is hemorrhaging, a door knocker is very hard to bang. I tapped. I slid my knuckles down the front of the wooden port.

Did I mention the freezing rain?

It took her a long time to get to the door. She looked annoyed. I was trying so hard to be a good girl, to avoid being sick or needy.

A man was in the kitchen; I was compelled to say hello, to shake his clammy hand.

The limo service was called, as was the chemotherapist, Dr. R. It was true. I was as pale as alabaster.

Things started to intensify when we got to Sloan Kettering. The whisk into the phlebotomy room. The seat outside the yellow hallway on the chemo side of the floor.

Marsha has done something wrong and is in A LOT of trouble, was the general consensus.

At least someone was paying attention to me.

I had a conversation with the Chassidic woman sitting next to me. She told me her husband was from Israel. He didn't speak much English. They had gone to a deli, where he had asked for "hard eggs." I thought that was funny. Out came Dr. R. He stood me up. It was a face-off. The yelling began.

"Do you know how dangerous your blood count is? You should be dead right now. Honestly."

A sixteen-year-old girl making an adult angry with her. Cool. "Your blood count is two. That means almost dead."

Two, huh? The sixteen-year-old girl was *sooooo* proud to still be standing, beating everybody.

The rest was not so fun. The cauterizing of my bladder, the constant scrutiny of my urine, the transfusions, and the overnights until my blood count was ten or higher, the missing out on schoolwork, on French, on friends. Two weeks into it I could not look at that gray wall one more day, or see yet another patient come and go.

First there was the girl with an eye tumor, constantly lying on her left side. She was in the left bed. She never wanted to talk. She was gone after I came back from some test. At least I had no chemo until the blood count improved.

What to do. Get better and jump right back into chemo, or stay sick at the hospital and feel trapped?

One night I heard a new roommate talking, she was in the bed on the left. She worked for *Interview*, like I even knew what that was. She was whispering to her girlfriend that she had had an abortion, her tumor was benign. She was released. She was lucky. No chemo. God loved her more than me, that was for sure. Plus, all those friends and family members were by her side constantly.

I read Tolstoy. And waited.

I was moved to the left bed. Almost time to leave!

My IVs infused, veins blowing. If one more infused, I could go home.

He picked me up, my dear father. As we crossed 69th Street to the parking lot (ugh, same street as Dr. R's cramped office), a car almost drove into us. My father hit the car with my paraphernalia-filled plastic hospital bag. He stood up for me.

I don't remember my mother coming to visit. I'm sure she did.

I have often equated success with financial status or career recognition. Honors. Interviews. Degrees. Competencies. Someone who contributed.

My mother always loved me in her own way. I think she is proud of me, but I have never known for sure. She should have held my hand through those four years. She should never have dropped me off and left me there, in a hospital bed, to throw up for hours, to have face-offs with forty-five-year-old physicians. She should have greeted me at the end of treatment, rather than call a limo driver to bring me back home to New Jersey. She should have noticed that I was slowly dying from a hemorrhage. She should have showed me that I was worthy. I guess she gave me what she could.

God's love is never haphazard. My mother's inattention has caused a great refinement in me. I am gold in the palm of His hand.

I am Mary's daughter.
In the morning, we work together, cleaning the house,
cooking the meals, watering the plants.
We laugh and sing.
She taps me on the head, then smiles into my eyes.

She is strict, demanding my attention, but she is so beautiful.
I love to be in her presence.
Her faith is earthy, well-seeded, outspoken, sometimes bawdy.

She hugs me often. She holds my hand tightly
as we walk through the market.
She is strong, soft, and proud. All the people
at the market adore her.
She shares honestly with others. She shows
me how to give with sincerity.

She sees in me a hidden talent—that of a soul knower.
She feeds me with strength. She trusts me.

She shares a secret with me that no one else will ever know.

Her sons and husband adore her, yet are slightly afraid
of her when she gives them her truth glance.
She expects to be respected. She expects me to be respected by her, as well.

She gives me permission to make huge mistakes
and welcomes me home no matter how far I have gone from her.
Her rhythm is constant, firm, and full of joy that I am here.
Even the smallest wound is met with tenderness by her.

She sees my path clearly and honors my ability to find it on my own.
She shows me how to live wisely and well.
She is involved in my life. I can count on her.
She equips me to be a woman of the earthenware god.
She teaches me every day that holiness is never separation. It is always
Unity.

CHAPTER 10

It is warmer in my heart today
And meaner on the outside
I am waiting for all the ugliness to go
And it does, in little pieces
I feel like I have no sweetness in my body right now
It is angry and sad everywhere
I miss the beautiful part of myself that has always been so shiny
Nice not to work so hard, though
I feel I still shine
Without all the effort
I am passing through something new
Old voice says hold on, hold on, hold on
New voice says open up, open up, open up
Get ready for the ride of my life
Open to my new ways
Amen.

I have a long history of righteous indignation. From the time they played a cruel trick on Janet during her fifth grade slumber party, to the moment my insurance company said I wasn't eligible for medical insurance, compelling me to drive to Senator Kennedy's office for clarification (which I got, along with a signed affidavit); I have been fueled by the desire to vindicate wrongs.

It came as no surprise that I applied to law school my senior year in college. I would save handicapped children, the disenfranchised of the globe. I would fight for the rights of all citizens to live freely, or else.

I was a very young twenty-one-year-old. Skinny, still a virgin, had never had a drink, the face of a teenager, scared of new places, worried about how much walking I would have to do to get to law school, armed with a degree in French and art history!

I had no clue what I was doing. I just knew I had to:

#1 Save the world.

#2 Meet a guy attending medical school, which was across the street from the law school.

All was going well until I actually went to class.

I studied diligently. Property law, constitutional law, torts (whatever they are), and contracts. Within a few weeks I was barely able to follow.

The professors helped keep my feigning interest. They had personas, compelling speeches, smirks on their faces, wildly gesturing arms, particular pacing techniques, fascinating clothing choices.

I spent a majority of my time trying to understand this one thing: why would one of the first female graduates of Harvard Law School, a dramatic, gorgeous woman with wavy hair and brilliance of mind running through her fingertips, be involved with "The Contract Guy"?

Granted, he was smart. Granted, he'd had great success in his career. But that potbelly? The disheveled jacket with the crumpled white shirt crushed underneath? Birkenstocks and bare feet in February? And the pièce de résistance: after he'd ask a contract law question, while looking at his chart to select a student, he would put one of his feet up on the desk and pick at his toes. Pick at his toes!!! Law school in the eighties was around ten thousand dollars a year. Ten thousand dollars for this? I prayed for his woman constantly.

By second semester I was furiously writing in my journal, longing for poetry and literature, French, Joan Miró i Ferrà, anything that was as far away from legal studies as I could imagine.

I did more than imagine—I ran off to a literature studies program, to spend a year in France, on a path toward a PhD in surrealism.

I chose Scotland for the summer. A six-week institute at the University of Edinburgh, to delve into Scottish and Irish classics. I was so happy. Late-night discussions of Scottish writers. Pub crawls with Spaniards who smoked too much. Classical guitar serenades on balconies from men named Michelangelo. The Fringe Festival. And my clothing, an anomaly in law school, was a huge hit in Edinburgh.

My deep pining in Scotland was nutrition-based. I tried to barrel through as much Weetabix as possible, because blood pudding and haggis were often on the menu. Greens and other vegetables seemed nonexistent, but scones with jam at least had "fruit" and butter . . . "protein." I managed to find the one Jewish bakery and restaurant serving healthy food close to town. I tried Italian once; the red sauce had mutton in it. I was so deprived that one day I bought a small, beaten-down green pepper and devoured it as if I were eating an apple.

Pneumonia came the fourth week. The director of the program didn't offer much advice or help. Leave it up to the Spaniards to pull through. They took me to the hospital, where I was prescribed penicillin—my first indication that I was allergic to the drug.

The doctor heartily declared that I was only experiencing a bout of pneumonia. Buckle up. Brace yourself. Have some haggis!

I went in and out of delirium all week. By Sunday, I was able to drag myself downstairs. The kitchen was closed. And although the cooks were there and could have easily cooked me at least an egg, they sternly informed me that they were off duty. Those damn Presbyterians.

If this had been Ireland, I would have had two eggs, brown bread, and a visit or two from the locals. Maybe even a pinch on the old arse. I retreated to the small TV room, where I spent the next few hours glaring at sheep races.

The following week my mother called from New Jersey: "The good news is, sweetheart, you got an A in property law. The bad news is, you failed law school."

The setup began. I had something to prove. Being alive in spite of . . . loving God in spite of . . .

Showing people God exists.

I felt I could do anything, despite all my health challenges and artificial leg. Buckle up. Brace myself. Don't complain. Eat some haggis!

I am not the one who will push you over
Trample you down
Make you afraid to stand
Or your turns uncertain

I am not the one who tucks into your ribs so you can't breathe
Who thinks he knows better than you
And drags you down with him

I am not the one who causes you to question your motives
They are sincere enough

I am not the one who doesn't know you
And makes your world unsafe.

I am the one who leads you
With true kindness
These hands of mine are trustworthy
They have built houses, countries, families, children

Eyes open
Eyes closed
I take care of you.
You can relax now.
And breathe.

Chapter 11

Jesus gave me a scripture. The word "stump" stood front and center.
Stump is a word I have never been able to say.
It is an ugly word.

Stuh

Ump

Like a bully,

Like a guttural woe,
Like no class,
Like low class,
Like cut off,
Like separate,
Like disgusting,
Like I am better than them,
Like I don't want to be them,
Like I don't want to be here, do I?
Like being here means a new trauma each week,
Like being here means I never get what I really want,
Like being here means I have no clue what I want,
Like being here it is selfish to want, when
so many are suffering every day.

I am twenty-five, so it makes sense to move to Los Angeles and open a hand-knit sweater company, with no background in business whatsoever, just because I like sweaters.

I design the sweaters, purchase the yarn, find the Korean knitters, get the wholesale license, and nab the fancy clients in New York City and LA.

A woman touches one of my angora sweaters. She says, "Mmm . . . who needs a boyfriend when you have this?" I am onto something.

Unfortunately, I have no clue how to run a business. The sweaters sure are pretty though.

I don't know how to fall in love. I dream of looking into my man's eyes as "La Mer" by Debussy is playing in the background. This happens in LA at least once. One night he doesn't show up. My next fellow says our relationship is too much like a movie. It is. I don't want to reveal anything too tough, but I do at least tell him I had cancer once. I leave out the bag on my stomach, the artificial leg. He just keeps commenting on the fascinating way I walk. I get drunk one night with him. I throw up. He kisses my head. We go to Big Sur. He kisses my mouth.

LA is not the ideal place to have a physical handicap. LA is okay with all the mental disabilities; those don't show up in head shots.

I met a man in LA at a party. His heart was so good, but it was a party, and I wanted to party in my twenties.

I was afraid to hug him, touch him, breathe near him. They knew so little then. I knew less. He was a friend of Michel's. Michel was the one I wanted to get to. There was that other girl, the Jersey queen.

Michel smoked pot all the time, and he was paranoid, but his eyes were so large and brown. He was seriously thinking about his Judaism. I wanted to know more. He had a red Ford Thunderbird circa 1967. We went to see Lou Reed. So French of him!

The man was interesting, questioning existence, life, and death. I was too entrenched in Bible-thumping Christianity and guilt to criticize my reasoning that he'd obviously done something wrong. I felt compelled to witness to him. He was open to even that. He was simply open.

And sick.

Very, very sick.

He kept talking about this disease, and his fear.

My friend Sophie had the wisdom to say, “He needs to speak.”

So I listened.

I don’t know if he made it. So many died out there in the mid-eighties. I still had a hard time with my rationale, considering rock stars who had slept with hundreds, if not thousands, of men and women, getting this horrendous disease. Weren’t they just a little accountable for their actions? What about all those little children dying from dysentery, malaria, and this dreaded disease simply by being born?

And then this man. Perhaps just a few partners, but still this disease, and surely a lot of suffering prediagnosis for being who he was.

WWJD?

I hate it when people tell me they’ve had their own personal Job experience. You can get back to me when you’ve endured all of Job’s tribulations at the same time, *plus* every disease possible: you stink, lose your house, lose all your children, lose your friends, lose your dog, don’t know whether to sleep or lie awake or kill yourself, and *still* won’t give up on God. We’ll talk then.

I complained to God one day.
“Lord, you ask so little of her faith.
She worries about how many friends she has,
Or whether her body is thin enough.”

“I know, but for her, it is very, very hard.”

I was peaceful.

CHAPTER 12

They also serve who sit and wait
for far too many hours
reading trashy magazines
watching bad television,
staring at other people's ill bodies in really unflattering hospital gowns,
horrible shoes, and excruciating fashion choices.

I have finally figured it out. Since this whole cancer/life-threatening almost all-consuming sickness thing started in 1967, I have clocked in an amazing thirty-seven thousand eight hundred and ninety-six hours (give or take a few) either waiting for a doctor's appointment, a surgery, an insurance broker, a medical test, a prosthetic appointment, a nurse, a tech, a weigh-in, or a medical procedure. Now that I am of a certain age, it appears I have accumulated more than four hundred thirty-five thousand four hundred and forty hours, or at least 13.82 percent of my life, on waiting around in a medical establishment for someone to call my name, poke, and prod me.

In the beginning, there were attempts at entertaining me with *Highlights* magazines, toys in the corner, coloring books, homework, fish tanks, songs, playrooms with overused games and sticky plastic chairs, people to stare at inappropriately, and scary clowns to visit me in my hospital bed. There were the better waiting rooms: rooms with cushy chairs, water coolers with buttons to press, books on kittens, soft carpeting, dim lighting, other kids, nice smells, and lollipops!
Mostly, though, the waiting has not been so pretty.

I used to wait at Dr. B's office, the one who rediagnosed me with bone cancer. His waiting room was beige. The chairs lined the edges of the wall, creating a huge space in the middle that would have been perfect for backflips and handsprings. But I had to sit still and WAIT! I had been waiting each year, from 1967, hoping that the cancer wouldn't come back. Every yearly checkup I would sit on his side of the office. The other side of the office was more interesting. There were more people coming and going and more maimed patients, as well as blue carpeting. Sometimes I would sigh loudly to irritate the other waiters, push my chair too close to another patient, pretend I had some strange twitching disease or a problem with drooling. ANYTHING to pass the time. The last time I went to Dr. B's office he had some bad news for me.

Too big, this information that I knew was coming. I waited in that office, fidgeting, restless, bored, bored, bored. I tried to do my homework, but I was worried, alone in the examining room, waiting. This time the sigh was real . . . and silent.

It's 1987. I had moved out to LA. While I was watching every calorie, intimidated by the mass of pretty, thin faces and bodies, a digestion conundrum began. Every time I ate or drank I experienced so much bloating that it became stressful; to consume too much food meant there would be consequences, like exhaustion, swelling in my fingers and toes, moving my belt more than two notches. I went annoyingly to a urine specialist.

There I sat in his office. His office was beigey blue, small enough for about a dozen patients to sit cozily. I hoped no one with bad breath would sit next to me. Blood tests, urine tests, and x-rays had been taken before my visit.

I sat in that waiting room talking to a woman who was waiting, too. One of my least favorite side effects of waiting in doctors' offices is other patients. She started to vent all about her truly terrifying health problems.

Her kidneys had already failed.

I didn't want to know.

She was sort of positive, a woman of dwindling faith.

I didn't want to know.

She had a mission: to help others with kidney disease.

Kidney disease? Is that what I had?

I DIDN'T WANT TO KNOW.

She seemed timid, yet strong.

She was what I would become years later as a patient on dialysis; the I-can-do-anything-even-though-dialysis-is-so-terrible-and-I-am-terrified patient.

There is something about kidney failure that is so dangerous, so much at the core of our health, our essence, that living with a broken kidney is really hard to grasp.

A major necessary organ is gone. A machine keeps you pumping, your blood visible outside your body for a full three to four hours. You meet that machine every other day for the rest of your life, or until further notice.

Why did this woman talk to me?

Was the doctor about to give me another death sentence?

Her positive outlook was a shroud, a cover-up for the anger and bitterness that consumed her. It was as if she wanted me to suffer, to feel guilty for not yet succumbing to kidney disease. I would understand her soon enough, but not that day.

The nurse called me into the office. The doctor told me my kidneys were functioning at 50 percent. They would eventually fail.

I was twenty-five. Kidney failure, if it really happened, was far-off, when I was "old," in my fifties.

The woman in the office said good-bye to me as I left. As I closed the door, I could hear her inner voice trying to latch onto me, like a dehydrated string I was supposed to drag around until I had suffered like her.

The string was a banner that said: "I need to know that I am not alone in this. I need to know that someone else will suffer this, too."

I went down to get a soda at the coffee shop, where I ran into Billy Idol. He was gorgeous, dangerous, and completely avoidable. But, hey, he checked me out and gave me that look of his. After a potential kidney failure diagnosis, he was the perfect angry badass antidote.

A year later I was on a date with Billy's architect. The architect had designed Billy's driveway, lined with studded rocks. Rock on!

Waiting room adventures are no picnic, but then again neither are picnics.

How many sob stories have I endured in waiting rooms? I have lost count. When people are waiting in medical offices, any fellow waiter becomes a captive empty well, apparently begging to hear every grotesque detail of their neighbor's medical conditions, their surgery dates, their terrible issues with the doctors, the hospital, or insurance. I have tried to be compassionate for so long, understanding that this waiting room may be the only time when a patient can truly be heard, unencumbered by family or medical staff.

But I don't want to hear it. I just don't. I don't want to hear about the day their life stood still or the day they had their wake-up call from God, the number of stitches their surgery required, the number of feces they emptied from their colon, or how they faint whenever they get a needle. Please! If I fainted every time I had a shot, would I even be writing this?

In one waiting room I saw a woman sobbing uncontrollably, her husband holding her for HOURS (while I sat alone, waiting to get another life-or-death terrifying test).The woman had been completely traumatized by getting one little eensy teensy needle. Wouldn't *that* be nice, to be held by your husband, to sob uncontrollably about a silly needle poke?

I didn't want to know what I know.

I don't want to relive my story or that of my fellow waiting room compadre. I don't want to hear anything negative about anything. I don't want to stay in the story of the survivor or the sick child or the constantly ill one. I want to be in the story of ME, whole, beautiful me: a dancer, a somewhat cute, silly, funny, fully ***alive*** woman.

There have been too many waiting rooms and too much waiting. Too many hours have been spent empty, uninspired, and alone, doing everything in my power to protect this precious cargo from the darkness around her.

This leads me to the obvious conclusion. Meditation is not for me. I have been in stillness for far too long. Stuck stillness. Sequestered stillness. Lonely stillness.

"Be where you are, empty your mind." *What have I been doing for the last forty years? Entertaining myself with waiting and being, I guess.*

Except for the polyester carpets, the overhead lighting, and all those medical smells: alcohol swabs, cold metal cabinets, bleach. Bleach covering up death. No windows. Needles in my arms so I wouldn't be able to move. Television reruns. No privacy. No vision of the outer world. Inner world is fine with me. I have had lots of opportunities to find it. Now I want OUT though. I have done my meditation. I have taken the deepest breaths ever. I have heard and seen it all.

I have more doctor's appointments in my future. I will attempt to use my time wisely. I will wait, sometimes two to three hours as the prosthetist fixes my prosthesis or the doctor finally shows up.

I am an adult now. No climbing up on the chairs, making silly faces, or fidgeting too much. Sometimes I amuse myself by seeing if my left fingers can wrap around my right ankle. I read and reread the labels on the cabinets. I will continue to accumulate my hours of waiting. If you see me in a waiting room, please rest assured I will not be listening to your retelling of your ingrown toenail surgery or your heart disease. I will be too busy waiting.

Chapter 13

When I first lost the use of my kidneys, they stuck
a protruding catheter, complete with blue plastic caps,
jutting out of my jugular on the right side of my neck.
It was August 1995 in Geneva, Switzerland.
What's a girl to do?

Detract and accentuate.

Hermès silk scarf wrapped neatly around the neck,
draping just so over my décolleté, tight black dress.
Massive Elsa Peretti silver ring glaring
from my right middle finger.
Chanel Coco Red lipstick.
Smile. Strut. Aaah.

The emergency plane ride back to NY was no exception.

Michel Klein wrap-style baby blue linen
skirt with a pleat down the front.
Matching baby blue linen jacket.
Lace cami.
Auburn curls cascading down my right side.
Givenchy cream satchel.

I couldn't stand up, but I sure looked good.

Silly guard at LaGuardia . . . Do you really think
I am carrying contraband in that overstuffed suitcase?
Oh, please don't touch my agnès b. see-through,
pale pink raincoat,
Or my navy quilted jacket from Galeries Lafayette.
Please don't mess up my red, clingy, three-button pima cotton shirt.
But he did.
Bastard!

I really wanted to shop at "the bargain shop of NY." I had been hearing about it from all my shopaholic friends in New York who would traipse off to Brooklyn or the Bronx or wherever "the great one" was located. All I knew was that it wasn't in Manhattan, so I couldn't get there. I waited until I moved to LA, where another was located. I could drive there instead.

I was new to LA and its various customs: the pastel suits, the overly tanned men and women; the skin pulled so tight I knew it couldn't even be pinched; the famous "I'd love to," which usually meant "unless a movie star, director, or agent gets me a better gig." I had nothing to offer but me. Apparently, that was seldom enough.

On another sunny, wimpy LA day in July, the hotter part of the year, when the smog sunsets are at their peak, I ventured out all by myself to the illustrious bargain shop. When I first entered the store, I couldn't decide whether it was really a clothing store or a fabric emporium. Everything was everywhere. The smelly, carpeted floor had obviously been trampled on for a number of years; I thought for sure I would find dangerous pins lurking deep within the folds of the rug. There was a cash register tucked within a linoleum-type contraption and operated by a gilded lady who was smothered in shimmery lipstick and intentionally bright pink stripes on her cheeks. Near her was a young Russian girl, drably dressed in beige jeans, an even plainer T-shirt, gray skin from years of oppression, and a glare the size of Milwaukee. I have never been to Milwaukee, so I am just guessing.

I walked through the store, not sure if it was better to leave to catch my breath or stay inside. Either way I was screwed, because there was no fresh air anywhere. I peeled back layers of clothing, price tags dangling from sundry items. I wasn't thrilled by what I saw, but it was *the store*; I'd heard so much about the amazing fare and the phenomenal prices, I wasn't going to give up. I found a few pairs of pants and a flowy shirt (that wouldn't be in style until 2002, but I am a Scorpio, and we always know trends way ahead of the rest of the world).

I found my way to the changing room, where I was pleasantly completely disappointed. Mirrors were everywhere. So were women. No privacy. And many of the women shared my Orthodox roots. I have never been able to change in front of an audience for the simple reason that I had seen a documentary on the gas chambers when I was a child.

Plus, there was the issue of my leg, the prosthetic leg that I kept so well hidden from the world. How was I going to change in front of all these strangers?

I placed my clothing choices on a bench in a corner of the room with less overhead lighting and angled mirrors. The flowy shirt looked okay, so that was good. Then came the moment when I had to pull off my pants. I did, shyly at first, but no one was looking. No one . . . until I tried on a pair of pants. I should have looked at them more carefully; the hem of the pants was very narrow, so I had to yank the pants over my prosthetic foot to pull up the pant leg. This was before I knew to bring a shoehorn with me. The pants were all right, a pale (pastel of course) green denim. I didn't like them. I didn't want them. I couldn't get them off my prosthesis. I would have to buy them.

One of the Jewish ladies in the dressing room noticed my struggle. She began to tug at the pants, but no luck. Finally, against every wish in my bones, I had to take off my prosthesis and continue trying to pry the pants off. No luck. But I had acquired broken nails and raw knuckles. It was simply awful. Another woman called in the manager, who promptly took my prosthesis, pants dangling to one side, no questions asked. For the manager, it was a matter-of-fact problem that had to be solved. I saw the manager wander through the entire store with my leg. What if she never came back? How would I ever walk again? She returned about thirty minutes later, saying the owner of the store had to use a tool, though she wouldn't specify which tool, to release the leg from the pants. I guiltily purchased the hideous pants, which had survived the ordeal unscathed, after getting dressed and thanking the manager and my new friends from the changing room.

God bless you bargain shop of LA. Many mitzvahs sent your way.

The heavy mantle
Of all I have done
To belong
To succeed
To matter
To stay here
To make a difference
Was thrown off today

I went to the sea
Made my prayers in the sand
Circled them with sticks and stones

The next day
I returned
A goose had walked the perimeter
Of the circle, in perfect line with the imprint I had left the day before
Then he had turned away, upwards in a gracious curve

Even he knew
My dreams are too important to be trampled upon

Chapter 14

Hospital Fashion Emergency Kit
To be best prepared for your surgery and recovery
Please be sure to bring:
Your attitude
A robe that accentuates your best assets
That can accommodate tubes, wires,
and uncontrollable bodily functions
Glitter spray
Inappropriate footwear
A tiara
A framed photograph of your secret lover
A copy of One Thousand and One Nights
That you place prominently on the lower corner of your bed
when all good looking doctors visit
Blush
A lace wrap that you casually drape over your left shoulder
Jazz playing on your radio
Two pink nonflammable candles
A bouquet of white roses
Lip gloss
A pocket mirror
Your favorite perfume
Your naughtiest smile

The first day I met my renal doctor at New York Hospital, I showed up in my black Chanel flats, fitted dress, and a new Hermès scarf. She looked me up and down. She was nearly the same age as I. We spoke in French, which was at least a little glamorous compared to what was going on around me.

As I left her office and pondered my new body with a GORE-TEX graft in my left arm, my very first thought was: I need to create a chic fashion line for dialysis patients, with snaps in just the right places.

My first few months on dialysis, I would show up in my velour leggings, purchased at Capezio in Paris, around the corner from the Opéra, my French, silk, white, button-down shirt, and three-inch heels.

The velour leggings stayed throughout my eleven years of dialysis. The heels and the white blouse had to go. Dialysis is a royal, bloody mess.

Out came the Patrick Kelly *"J'aime Paris"* T-shirt with the wide sleeves. Add a little black belt and I could be going anywhere—just not to *that* place.

But I was there all the time.

When I got to Massachusetts, I switched to fitted, short-sleeved T-shirts, short shorts or flowing skirts, ballet flats, and long, dangling earrings. I added essential oils. I carried an amber stone that I placed on the corner of the table.

The day I was admitted to the hospital for my bladder reconstruction, I showed up in a linen, above-the-knee Anthropologie wrap dress. The doctor thought I was a hottie. Mission accomplished!

I wore my yellow, Swiss dot, Christian Dior robe and nightie, which was pretty fun to get in and out of with a multitude of tubes hooked to various parts of my body. But I looked good when I traversed the hallways after surgery.

The day I left the hospital, the wrap dress would not fit, so I draped it over my green hospital pants. My hair was pulled back. I wore makeup, which barely covered the obvious signs of malnutrition on my face. Still, I wore makeup.

The day I got my kidney, it was all so rushed. I did not have time to get my outfit together, not even grab my "ready-for-transplant" red leather satchel, complete with makeup bag, special brush, hand-knit booties (no hospital booties for me), and new nighties with plunging necklines in silky fabrics. My hospital fashion emergency kit.

After the transplant, my frequent hospital visits for the first six months provided the few opportunities I had to be fashionable. Fitted tops, slenderizing skirts. Granted my budget had changed. Givenchy was replaced with Target. There is always a way to "make it work."

I have already planned my outfit for my funeral. Yves Saint Laurent original black dress, black silk stockings, red garter belt. Givenchy low black heels. Nails in pale pink. Coco Red lips. Kohl eyeliner. My hair spread out along the pure silk white coffin interior, like the Shri goddess that I am.

I may be dead, but I'll look really good.

Just one little word
A song to be sung
Just one little voice
And no bells to be rung

Want more than was given
Want more than enough
Want all fears forgiven
Want sweeter, less tough

Just one little word
One pause in the story
Just one little voice
A song without worry

A day without fear, fear, fear
A new kind of feeling, a new kind of year

I'll get it. I'll have it.
It will be mine.
I'll see it. I'll know it.
I'll step over the line.

Just one little word
A new song is sung
Just one little voice
A new bell is rung.

Chapter 15

Good morning siren
Blazing red and gold
Into my ears and eyes
You have pierced me
In the tropical winds
On a balcony
By the grayness of a crowded city
Near the open air
And the coyote's loud cry of hope
I hope in you
The breath you bring
Your fire
Inside me
Wild, untamed
Following me
From city to city
Heart of flesh and fire
Siren
I hear you
I am coming to make you my own

I started to dress beyond my sexual means when I moved to Los Angeles. Everyone was beautiful there, so it was difficult to stand out and get noticed. You get the picture.

I was twenty-four. Very virginal. Very Christian. Eternally optimistic. Continually questioning my desirability factor.

I was always yelling at God about why He made me a Scorpio if he didn't want me to be totally satisfied. Not meeting a man was His fault.

I was overdressed. My weapons of choice: a touch of Audrey Hepburn class mixed with blouses cut too low, pouty red lipstick, masses of black cascading curls, skinny legs too long for my torso, and blue Irish eyes anointed with 1965-style black painted eyeliner.

My day, and hence my existence, was never complete unless oodles of good-looking men stared me up and down, while I coyly pretended not to notice. It never occurred to me to smile and say hi. I assumed that was their job.

At home, NEVER out in public, I would stare at my inspired Frenchish outfit, my body, and my smile.

I would drop down into my worry world, pretend to have it all, and then greet the day and the men with this strange sense of my inherent value based on male attention. Even though I was a Christian and knew better.

My accomplished day also required that lots of women gave me dirty, jealous looks, which meant I was really gorgeous and able to attract any man I wanted.

This all took a lot of work.

I even had a tape measurer to make sure my waistline never exceeded twenty-four inches.

I took an abs class, loaded with men, at the local Y. The janitor used to shout out "OWWW! Here comes dangerous." They all noticed, these guys, but I never helped them along. Let them do the work. I've done my part.

Too bad I had no clue what to do with a man once I got one!

He was always spouting wisdom
He said she would not listen

She exploded around him

*A whisper here—**you** cannot dance with fire says he*

"I am everything that holds you together"
He lifted his eyelid
Distracted
By
Something

She had already spun the world into Being.

CHAPTER 16

I am that piece of dust
That never seems to go away
I come back
Though you brush me off
I AM the woodwork
I do not fade
I do not fade
I do not fade

The year is 1987. It is dry in the desert as I walk past roadrunners, brush, and dirty sand in the road. A woman comes along the quiet, empty road to smile, laugh, and inspire me. I am on my way to a tiny Catholic church set back from the road. The woman walks this desert road to and from work every day. She leaves me at the church. I think she might be an angel. I enter the church. I stay for hours.

After passing the California licensing exam for teaching, I get a job as a teaching assistant. I spend a year in the hot, sunny classrooms. LA has become a place of such profound unhinging. It is not my imagination. It is also not all my fault.

There is nothing hearty about the relentless sun, imported palm trees, or green lawns where only sandy dirt should be. I am unmoved by the drug addict producers, the alcoholic actors, the sleazy, false power that only not-hard-earned money can buy. I feel lost in a world (as one should) where the next best thing is the next best person to use or disuse. Everybody has an angle.

I have too much flow for this place. I decide to get my masters in teaching.

I go to the desert one last time. I hit a place in the reserve where the sand and stones can drop into oblivion from the torrential downpours during rainy season. The sign says, SUBJECT TO FLOODING.

I can no longer live in a place where brief showers are so overwhelming.
I must go home soon.

But first the doctor tells me, "It is only a matter of time before your kidneys will fail."

We'll see.

I wait and don't wait at the same time. That is always the way. Never a question.

LA can make a person of substance want to do something more meaningful. I dream of Harvard. So I get in. I walk on ice in March, just to get to class. I am sure I will meet the man of my dreams at Harvard. I eat a lot of tofu. It's cheap. I learn how to respect everyone's opinion. It is so irritating.

List of grievances:

Lack of answered prayers, I forgive you.
People saying God always answers your prayers, I forgive you.

Hopelessness and desperation when prayers
aren't answered, I forgive you.
Forcing myself to believe that my prayers are
and have been answered, I forgive you.

Shame on you, jealous girl. God obviously loves
her more than you. Her prayers are answered,
I forgive you.
Miracles—why does He perform them so
often for the ones who haven't chosen him,
what's that about? I forgive you.

Lack of miracles—why does He deny them
so often to the hurting, helpless ones. What's that about?
I forgive you.

I don't trust you very much, forgive me.

Men who have harmed, the mothers,
the fathers, cruelty, sisters and brothers, friends,
the guy at the gas station, the woman
cutting in front of you in line, the liars,
the cheaters, the stealers, the child hurters,
the charmers, the wiseasses,
the arrogant, the selfish, the sneaky,
the ones who have too much
and don't share, the copiers,
the nasty girls, the false prophets,
the despots, the tyrants, the uberneedies,
the boundaryless, the cold, the heartless, the ruthless,
the ones who should be grownups but aren't,
the until-something-better-comes-along types,
spring coming too soon, heat and humidity,
not being allowed to live, the abusers,
the one who slammed the door in your face,
the abandoners, the less-than-up-fronters, the devaluers,
the ones who get away with it, I forgive you.
I am all that, too. Forgive me.

I love you, body. You are the walking breath
of God. You are GOLD in the palm of His hand.
Forgive Him.
It all started with a cell. I forgive you.

What followed . . . there is nothing to forgive.

CHAPTER 17

The doctor gave me six months before my kidneys would fail.

Here is what my "friends" told me at church:

Consider it a personal challenge.
It is God's will.
Stop complaining.
Be grateful to be alive.

"But is it okay to want just a little more?"
whispered my fading heart.

It is fine to be angry at God

. . . until I expressed my anger. Then I heard

God is hurt by your anger.

OKAY THEN.

Paris here I come.

I pack so many suitcases, including an empty one, fully intending to come back to the states with lots of French loot, including a thick-lipped, muscular, French spouse. I have a romance right before I leave with Gregory Peck, Latvian style.

I drive Madame Gely, my landlady, crazy. Her mumbling is so thick that I pretend not to hear that I can't cook in her kitchen. She is flabbergasted when I show up one day with cauliflower and millet. I sneak a rose into her bedroom every week. She is mortified, but she cries when I leave.

I am bored with simply going to the Sorbonne. I want some cash, so I go through the inane, utterly depleting, demoralizing paperwork of a student/work permit. I have no idea where to go, so to spite the ever spiteful French bureaucracy, I actually complete every annoying form needed.

After ensuring it isn't a famous saint's birthday, and being certain to avoid offices that were on strike, I wound up in the 9th quarter. There is *one* clerk (who proved to be a jerk) and no one else in the office, so, naturally, he pretends I am not there. I've got his number.

We are nowhere near lunchtime, a coffee break, or an official holiday.

Eventually Frenchy asks me what I want. My leg is tired and blistered. After limping through the streets of Paris, where some French people actually mimic my limp or point at me laughing, I am ready for this one.

He gloats, "You must go to another location to pick up blah blah blah form." Blah blah blah is an overused phrase in France.

"Do you mean this one?" I reply meekly.
"Well, this won't do without an EEU passport," he retorts.
"Do you mean like this?" I say, as my Irish passport emerges from my Roots knapsack.
He sighs deeply.

I do not go back to the 9th while I am in Paris. Within a week, I am legally teaching English. I take the two subways and long train out to Orly. I always forget to pack a lunch, but there is an Ovaltine machine. While it is of no interest to me whatsoever, I learn all the parts of an airplane so my mechanic students can properly learn English. Out of complete boredom, I decide to play hangman and Concentration with grown French men. My students improve their English dramatically over the course of the year. I even have dinner with some of their families. I eat too much baklava and play Trivial Pursuit in French. I get all the political questions wrong. But, then again, I would in any language.

I meet a friend in Paris. She is American. We dream of getting an apartment together. I move back to NYC, where I break up with my gorgeous Latvian.

What to do, what to do?

I know! I'll get my PhD in French.

Soon I am climbing the stairs to the fifth floor of Philosophy Hall at Columbia, immersing myself in deconstructionism and medieval triptychs and scarfing down free cookies at afternoon tea.

I never ever have a proper job. I have vocations, invocations, prayers, feelings, inspirations. I get by.

I live in Germany because any good PhD student should know German.

I try to like the country, but clearly this is not France, and we are not speaking French. I manage to live in a house with my own shower and loft. I love it, but it is miles from the school, and the fellow students, including some cutie-pie Italians. The jasmine petals flood my path every day. Little clowns and china trinkets line windows in the quaint Bavarian town that also houses a torture museum. I buy Japanese noodle soups.

I get pneumonia, like I always do when I go to a foreign country alone. I can't wait to leave anyway. I spend more than two hundred dollars on a phone call to a friend in NYC.

The kidneys are trying very hard to stay afloat from the 1980s to 1995. Their buoyancy is fading. I find a way. I must. I don't go to church much anymore. Everyone wants to pray for me, but they also don't want me to be negative. God forbid.

Repair Re-Pair Re-appear Re-Pear

Delphine was cooking poached pears soaked
in wine when we arrived at Sophie's house in Toulon.
I almost fainted. I mean, who in the
US makes poached pears for an evening snack?
More like popcorn in the microwave.
***I** would make poached pears soaked*
in wine, drizzled in chocolate,
on Friday nights when I returned to New York.
***I** would eat croque monsieurs instead*
*of grilled cheese. **I** would place*
my knives on knife rests.
***I** would lounge around on white shag rugs*
while I leaned my right elbow on a tufted cushion,
all the while laughing and holding
my wine glass in my right hand.
***I** would sip my coffee dosed heavily*
with sugar and milk from a simple ceramic bowl.
***I** would casually tie my scarf around*
my pocketbook when I walked through the city.
In France, everything counts.
So would I, one day.
Sophie placed me in a room
on the top floor of her family's home.
The sea was so close, the wood
furniture sticky with dampness.
I was here in France with Sophie,
but somehow I had managed to leave
parts of my body suspended in space.
Sophie came in to explain the toilet to me.
I pretended to understand, shaking my head yes.
Let's be clear: the moment someone
explains anything technical to me,
I have already stopped listening.
This time, Sophie caught me in the act.
"Why are you nodding yes
when you don't understand?"
I couldn't agree more.
By the end of the weekend,

the toilet was mastered,
but I had still lied to my friend.
Sophie took me to an island.
We hiked to the top.
There, she shared with me the echo
of the ocean waves on the shells,
unique to the Côte d'Azur.
I tried to hear but I had no reference point.
Why is it that now I remember
that sound more than any other experience in France?
Sophie was like that, climbing
to the tops of hills and such,
hearing the sounds of the ocean,
the wind in trees indigenous to the land,
holding a tiny seed in her hand,
amazed at its shape and texture.
She flipped her thick blond hair often,
especially with men around.
She laughed all the time.
This is Sophie, and this is also France,
where beauty is life itself.
I wish America were like that.
America saved my life. France saved my soul.

CHAPTER 18

Forgive yourself for your doubt. It is only natural.

I became a squirrel gathering food
before winter. There was little left.
Forgive yourself for your fear. The needles
are sharp. The body is protecting.
I became a dog who ran away from
the vet every chance he got.

Forgive yourself for your anxiety.
Who was going to get you out of that mess?
I became a seal trapped in a fishing net.

Forgive yourself for your sadness.
You were never meant to be alone.
I became the infant eagle whose mother had died.

Forgive yourself for your envy. You had a right to play too.
I became a cat rubbing its body against
someone's leg, only to be kicked away.

Forgive yourself for your anger. This wasn't your dream.
I became a pit bull forced into the killing ring.

Forgive yourself for your insecurities. It is wobbly out there.
I became the seed attempting to replant
in soil after the volcano has erupted.

Forgive yourself for your resentment.
You were only trying to understand the impossible.
I became a woman who had desires.

I went to the resentment cell
to find His love. And to forgive Him.

One day, while I am in my PhD program, I decide I must do something more meaningful.

Within a few days, I have an appointment with a director of children's programs at the UN. By summer I am living in Geneva, witnessing revolts against genetic engineering in food, and interning at the Center for Human Rights. My dream summer! Europe. An internship at the UN. The Alps as a backdrop. A clock made of flowers gracing a bridge over Lake Geneva, which told me if I would be late for a session or not.

It is tough to walk to the UN. I want to do things with the other interns, but I don't want to tell them I have an artificial leg. My summer started out wonderfully, except for the looming kidney song, "When will they fail? They better not fail. They will not fail because I have faith. Do I have enough faith? They are going to fail because I don't have enough faith."

Fashion inspiration. Smoldering, barely shaven men with foulards, thick, wavy hair, and way too much cologne. Although I was not much of a Calvinist myself, what with all the joyless rules and endless work ethic that was supposed to bring us salvation someday, I lived at the women's home that had, at the height of Calvin's heyday, been a women's home for Calvinist devotees. His dry, uneventful-looking church was across the street.

I had an equally dry, uneventful single room overlooking the tip of an old rooftop. I shouldn't say completely uneventful. Sometimes laundry hung from a tiny attic window, and how they got those flowers into the flower beds up there was remarkable. My bed was more like a cot. The room and the city were sweltering, with no ice cube in sight. We were only offered breakfast; a meal I never eat.

We could not use the main kitchen to cook our meals, and, of course, there were no markets close by. We all stuffed whatever food we could find into one refrigerator on the third floor. I bought a cheap pot and mostly ate spaghetti with olive oil and olive bread dipped in olive oil, thanks to the only bakery within walking distance of the Calvin home (which was disdainfully considered a place for way-too-independent women).

I also ate too much chocolate. There was chocolate everywhere.

Famous, epicurean-grade chocolate shops were as numerous as delis in Manhattan. If I could not find a decent vegetable or fruit without spending a fortune on a meal, I could indulge in a fistful of praline crème milk chocolate shaped like swans, pillows, or the Swiss flag.

Those were the days of the "old leg"—the one that caused blisters if I walked too many miles. I walked too many miles every day. I didn't want to miss a thing. I couldn't. I wandered the streets of Geneva searching for chocolate.

Baywatch is great education when you have nothing to do in Geneva. Dubbed in French or *suisse allemande*, it was easy for me to practice my foreign languages. Women outrageously unclad, rushing into the water to save helpless hot men, women, children, and more hot men. Simple phrases, limited vocabulary. America indeed! I had never seen the show before living at the Calvinist home for way-too-independent women. I often returned from another inspiring day at the UN, shortened by my exhausting limp, to straddle the faded, sheet-covered armchair propped in front of the community television. I could hang out with women who, like American college girls following a soap opera, would gather to create commentary, criticize American imperialism or bad fashion sense (I can't remember which created more friction).

Oh how I wanted to take off that LEG! But my sweltering, blank-walled room, with the few sprigs of lavender, was not beckoning me.

Even in Geneva I thought, sometimes I am so embarrassed to be labeled an American. How much time could a girl spend watching French-dubbed American television with really bad acting? I would eventually go upstairs to dip my olive bread in my olive oil and listen to really good eclectic music. At least there was a radio in the room. I should have been having a lot more fun.

The Chinese herbs didn't help, either. I drank this concoction of brown muddy herbs every day. I had a thermos full of the stuff. It was supposed to ward off the impending kidney failure. But it was not chocolate!

Every day I went down to the UN café at 10:00 a.m., again at around 2:00, then 4:00, and, of course, it being the UN and Europe and all, the workday was over by 7:00. Time for cocktails. I wandered the UN halls like a queen, sneaking into hidden libraries, dusty caverns, and unused offices, discovering papers in foreign languages and metal bins filled with more piles of stuff than I had ever seen. I watched demonstrators outside the UN gates. I took buses around the city to lectures at the Red Cross, humanitarian gatherings, leisurely lunches. I heard every language being spoken, every culture represented. The organic markets, the Goth art houses were everywhere.

Every day I walked down the hill from my hostel. Every day I passed the small shop that sold my olive bread and the café with lukewarm Limonata. I passed the carousel, the ice cream stand, the elegant (not nearly as fashionable as Paris)shops and crossed the bridge. I was supposed to live here, to become a UN employee and an artist and meet a gorgeous European man and live like Audrey Hepburn in a château and take ballet classes and become a yogi. I was supposed to do this.

The message always slithered in from my right side, "Your kidneys will fail . . . and soon. You will never get your dreams." So I worked harder at pretending I felt fantastic. I went out when I could, trying hard not to limp or appear sick in any way. The Spaniards seem to get the partying thing so well. I just couldn't drink that much without getting truly ill. So I was quiet. I dove into D. H. Lawrence and prayed for my gatekeeper. I didn't get a gatekeeper, but a real cutie-pie who made out with me beneath Monsieur Calvin's church bells. He told me I needed to stop eating *les pâtes* (pasta). Tell me about it. God, I just wanted some protein. He was an almost good substitute, for a minute.

A friend of my sister's lived over the border in France. She was someone I could connect to while I was there. (More like someone who would watch over me!) She had a phenomenal job at the UN. Her laugh was large.

So were her breasts, filled with milk. She would nurse her baby in public, at the town café where she lived; she knew it irritated the patrons, which made her more determined.

I need a Soldier.

I'll go!

NO!

Oh. This is so . . .

beautiful.

CHAPTER 19

I opened my altar.

I went into the inner chambers of the soul.
The wounds were plentiful.
A soldier tortured over
and over for fighting injustice.
His supposed contract?
"I have to fight. It is my eternal duty."
He walked atop the smoky rubble,
a helmet tight around his head, his breath constricted.
Angels came to lay him down on
a soft bed. They lifted a pale pink
blanket up to his chin. Rest!
I looked in the mirror. He spoke,
"NO MORE BATTLES."
The water poured down through
the aqueducts of tears, belly, heart, throat, Spirit.
Peace Descended.

He has given me a new contract.
A wave is seldom disappointed.
Or indignant. I think I'll stay.

Two days before it all went down, before the rescue and the sunflower episode, I sat down at the café around the corner from my hostel. It was just after work, maybe 2:00 p.m. I saw *the* most gorgeous man sitting at another table. I had on my Donna Karan black dress, the one with the fitted top and full skirt. My thick, wavy hair was pulled up in a loose chignon. I pretended not to notice the man as I unraveled my bun, in more ways than one. I sighed as I did this, looking demurely toward the ground. I got up and walked away, giggling inside because I knew he had seen me, knew his jaw had dropped. He followed me. I pretended to be annoyed.

He took me to another café—like I really wanted another lukewarm drink. Adel, Arabic for light, was from Egypt. We agreed to meet the following night for dinner. The next day I followed my usual route down the cobbled sidewalk. I got as far as the carousel. I could not take another step. I found my way to a phone. My sister's friend took me to her house.

It was only the flu, right? Of course I had not gone to the bathroom in a month. Of course my head was on fire. Of course my midback was rounded over. I lay on the floor in a small overheated apartment in France, listening to Björk. By nighttime I was at the French hospital.

It was only constipation, right? Two, three saline enemas later, there was nothing. It is only an infection. Take some penicillin. My sister's friend found a twenty-four-hour pharmacy in the middle of a gray French suburb.

Within an hour, the anaphylactic shock set in. A miraculous decision was made. "This is no job for France," reasoned my sister's friend, "I am taking you to Switzerland."

More enemas. More nothing.

"I only need to walk."

They let me walk barefoot through the halls; I wouldn't put those hospital "shoes" on my feet. If I did, it would be official—I was sick.

After the allergic reaction to penicillin, the countless blood tests, the myriads of medical interviews in French (Who knew that I'd mastered the French medical lingo?), my beautiful doctor came in to see me. Something new—besides the fact that he was yet another elegant, handsome European man. He leaned his back against the white wall, then slid down to squat, hands folded at his bent knees, his voice soft like a father's. "Marsha, *vos reins ne marchent plus*." Your kidneys don't work anymore.

My throat dropped into my heart; I could no longer speak. How to get back—how to get back to my body. Chills set in all along the tiny hairs on the skin. The heart drew in to close the circuit of stepping out of the fear. *Stay, Marsha. Stay.* Everything swirled in my head. I tried to find my hands. Oh, this is all so familiar.

I didn't notice at first that the doctor was crying. His tears calmed me immediately. He explained what would happen the following day. Words that ran by me rather than through me. I was trying to find the fear in my body and hold onto it for dear life. Fear = Alive!

Switzerland is a very good place to have a serious illness. The doctors cry. When you ask for water, the nurses bring a glass bottle of Perrier in a silver bucket filled with ice. The sheets are 100 percent Italian pima cotton in a faded blue with peach highlights. Your hospital room has a balcony from which you can do Tai Chi facing the Alps. They don't put IVs in until it's completely necessary. The yogurt that comes with your meal is made from local Swiss cows. Television channels include programs from other nations, news that includes the WORLD.

Handsome men named Adel rush to your side to hold your hand, cry, and teach you Arabic. Nurses run down the hall after handsome men named Adel leave, giddy with excitement that such a movie star gorgeous man would be visiting one of their patients. Patients casually reply, "Oh, he is just a friend." A friend who writes letters to you in French for years, always ending with "*Je pense à toi tout le temps.*" I think of you all the time.

I ran away from the hospital the morning after my arrival, desperate to have one more day on the outside before my imprisonment. I thought freedom wouldn't come until I was much older—in my forties!

I didn't know if I would come back. I mean, what would be the harm in dying young on a sidewalk in a small town outside Geneva? Then my older question crept in. When would I *ever* get to live a life without fear? The twelve o'clock sun was much too bright. I worried that I had not put on my sunscreen. Ridiculous!

The sunflower field appeared on my right. I don't know how many miles I had walked. Thousands of bright yellow faces blew in the wind. I paused, tears rolling down, but I did not feel them. My roots rose up. I turned around.

Frantic nurses and doctors scrambled around me upon my return, furious I had left the hospital. An intern came to jam a catheter down my jugular, without anesthesia, into the cavity inside my heart. He poked and poked. I choked and choked.

Several hours into the night, every cell was shaking with new memories. In the morning, they wheeled me to the dialysis room. I saw *that* lounge chair waiting for me. My breath shortened. My fingers lost sensation. The warm, smiling nurse welcomed me. I collapsed in the middle of the floor.

"*Ça va bien, chérie. Ça va bien.*" All is well, my darling. All is well. She set me up in the lounge chair, tucking me in with a warm blanket and some hot chocolate. All sweet and smiling as she connected a tube to the catheter in my neck. Within three hours I felt better than I had in years. There was a window in the left-hand corner of the room. I knew they were out there, the sunflowers. And I was in here, choking.

I frantically searched for alternatives.
I did EVERYTHING—macrobiotics,
acupuncture, yoga, meditation,
colonics, herbs, holistic doctors, Tai Chi, Ayurveda.
I am a fighter, after all.

I know! I'd write a cookbook
for kidney patients, one that keeps them off dialysis.
I could beat this. I had faith. Besides, God loved me. Smile.

Clearly, that day in Switzerland
when my kidneys went south, I had failed, failed, failed . . .

Chapter 20

This is my body.

This is my body on trauma.

These are the scars of my body.

Here is a map of my scars.

If you want to talk about holding onto a thread for dear life, come to a dialysis unit. The thread is a plastic tube, pulling really dirty blood out from a lifeline (fistula or graft) and pushing clean-ish blood back in. My threads were *anything* that nourished my spirit, since nourishment from food and water was inconsequential.

I taught that dialysis a thing or two about what constitutes life force. I still hated it. Oh how I hated it. My heart was broken by this half-life. I wanted more.

This forced, exiled rest was ugly. Overhead lights beamed down. Buzzers sounded all around me. Sickly, nervous people sat nearby. People were stuck in their recliners, all part of the big blood-cleansing factory.

Hate is not a word I come to lightly. Eleven years of these dialysis shenanigans gave me cause to hate. I hated dialysis.

I was grateful, because it kept me alive—but still, I hated it. I hated seeing the diabetics with their missing limbs and blind eyes. I hated witnessing the comatose elderly, wheeled in on stretchers. I hated observing the puffy-eyed, gray-skinned, morbidly obese who looked like they hadn't taken care of themselves a day in their life. I grieved the short-statured thirty-to-forty-year-olds who had lived with kidney disease their whole lives.

I hated being there.

I hated the kindness dance I felt I needed to do with doctors and nurses because I had to see them three times a week. I hated the false camaraderie, born of so much misery. I hated this teetering between life and death, as precariously close as a plastic tube with my blood running through it visible to my naked eye.

There is a moment during the dialysis life, where giving up seems like the right thing to do. It is at that moment one has to decide whether he or she is worthy of life or not.

It happened for me about ten years into it. I sat at the edge of the chair, after another close encounter with a medical terrorist. I was deciding: cry, don't cry? How much more, Lord? How much more? It is the first time a nurse was worried about my emotional state. Usually I walked into and out of that unit with a smile, and not a fake one, either, now I know. It was the first time I honestly lied to a nurse about how I was feeling. "No, I am fine." Just don't ask me to say one more word.

Have you ever taken a tour of a dialysis center?

Why would you?

A typical dialysis room is a big blank room with nonstop buzzers and beepers, overhead lights, no privacy, cold floors, blood spills, overwhelming smells of bleach, lounge chairs feigning cleanliness (don't look in the crevices where all the blood congeals), and a whole bunch of technicians running about (often to handle the threat of a patient's low blood pressure).

Unless I was confined to the dialysis chair, I seldom sat down.

Today I am forced to sit; I take off my prosthesis and sling it onto the shelf behind the beeping machine. It is cold in here, and I am naked beneath my ratty fleece blankets. I have weighed myself. Only three kilos gained since my last treatment. Perhaps I will get through my session without cramping, perhaps I won't crash this time, perhaps I won't have to hope some nurse or tech gets to me in time to flip me upside down before I clot my graft, fistula, or neck catheter.

I am careful to not reveal the packet of Cheez-Its and Reese's Peanut Butter Cups I snuck in.

How are they going to plant those 14mm needles in my arm? Why, ethyl chloride spray, of course! Nurses be damned. A moment of shortened breath comes before the needle meets my skin, and my four-hour journey into restlessness begins. I can't move much, as I might dislodge a needle or cause a cramp in my calf. Sleep happens occasionally, amidst the overhead lights, the scurrying nurses, and the fervor of the occasional emergency.

One old lady died next to me. She, who had spoken not a word in years, asked the nurse for her brush. Right after she fixed her hair for God, she was gone.

By hour three I am back in my mind, willing myself not to cramp or crash. I focus with all my will on talk shows or bad Christian TV (Why did God heal so many people other than me?) and try to stay relaxed. If I make it, I am usually blood pressure-depleted. I pop my ears, move my jaw, swallow, wait. The needles come out. I press hard on the now-tiny wounds. Sometimes there are blood explosions and messy fingernails, even blood spatters on my face, blanket, or T-shirt. I have lost the need to feel dirty about this, I just want to get home. I reach behind me for my prosthesis. I slide it on, along with my pants. If all goes well, I am three kilos less until the next treatment. I pack my things, get to the car, and drive home.

The weekends demanded an extra dose of willpower. Drink even less, eat even blander, sweat more, do too much. Fend off. Fend off. Fend off.

I decided to take my first trip, to see if I could. I told the nurse coordinator I wanted to go to Beverly Hills, figuring they'd have a nice dialysis unit there. I got my rental car, checked into my rockin' hotel (where the staff thought I was part of a heavy metal band; who was I to disagree?), and set out for treatment.

As I approached South Central LA on Beverly Boulevard, a gated dialysis unit glistened from across the police station. Isis nursed me. When I grew cold, she covered me in paper sheets (all they had), told me I was bright and beautiful, practically mauled me with love.

I awoke to rattling chains and a string of the most handsome, fit black men I had ever seen. Prisoners. Here for dialysis. How much more chaining can one endure? Maybe dialysis, for them, represented a type of freedom.

I have to make a room just for hopelessness today.
Drooping Leaf
Listless Spirit
Exhausted Heart
Depleted Soul
I have to make a room for these,
the unwanted parts.

I cling to oxygen, but the branches are dwindling.
The Tree is slowly dying from roots to crown.
I know I am the "vibrant once" trying to maintain,
trying to maintain,
So tired.

Heart wants to hope but the blood,
the blood is so thin
I lift up my middle finger,
to let the world know I am still around
Courage, bravery, strength,
Power.

I am straddled on the lounge chair
made to look so comfortable
I have never been comfortable there

I am holding up the hope for all of us
I just want a moment when I can refrain
from apologizing for wanting to give up
A moment where I can allow death in,
regardless of what they need
I just need a moment of sustained silence
Reverence for my inability to take in any more suffering
A moment of grace
A moment when I don't know if it will ever pass
A moment of long, deep caving in
Without this moment there is only partial resurrection
Be full of your hopelessness, He says
Let me dive in there with you
It is just a room like any other

In my Father's house there are many rooms
I was alone in the room with my hopelessness,
Until it was completed,
My death.

I go to the room often now
My only way to be alive again,
Resurrected beyond measure
This great thing have I accomplished in my life:
I have made a room for hopelessness,
and entered it willingly.

Chapter 21

I thought it would be fun to light a red candle
and meditate on the undomesticable feminine.
I had nothing else to do that night.

Moments into finding her, I began to sob.
I saw her dancing red body, red arms flailing.
She held my prosthesis between her teeth, tearing it apart,
gnashing at it, head thrashing from side to side.
She was SO angry my roots had been taken away from Her,
cutting off my firmness to Her ground.

I heard myself singing.
La la la.
Hissing.
Lie lie lie.
Crying out.
Life, Life, Life.

The day I was able to avoid shutting off the valve of my heart completely was the day I was honest.

God gave me a rose for that.

The woman I met at the photography workshop on Lexington Avenue was tall, brown, a model (I think), and fluid in her sexuality. I had finally gotten out of my cloistered apartment, away from my desk, my French literature, my windows overlooking the barren tree with the plastic garbage bag dangling from one of its branches.

I got away from chain-smoking Stella, my neighbor, who, although elegant like Audrey Hepburn, was covered in a cloud of raspy fumes accompanied by a raspy voice. Still, her little low black heels and skinny jeans made an impression.

I escaped the grumpy writer sequestered in the bungalow behind me who would later win a Pulitzer.

The photography workshop took place at the 92nd Street Y.

There, at the 92nd Street Y, I found a world other than the small, stuffy with ego arena I was crammed into day after day.

One night I attended a lecture, offered by Anna Deavere Smith and Jane Alexander, about the National Arts Council. Handsome Charlie Rose dashed by me like an intellectual gust of overstimulating air, along with his entourage.

The Y gave me back my dance on the night I signed up for Afro-Cuban dance. I took off my shoes, stepped onto the floor, and began to move with the rhythm of the drums. The teacher imparted life in each step, reminding us to walk around like we owned the place.

Oil painting grabbed my interest for one hour, but, as I expected, required me to understand angles, planes, horizons. Oh, how tiresome.

The Y introduced me to photography.

It wasn't that I was particularly good or "ungood." Photography was a way I could finally express my black-and-white feelings for life in New York and the impending kidney failure without hurting someone, including myself.

The class was only ten blocks from my apartment. In the winter, with slick sidewalks, traffic, and crowds, the ten blocks could be treacherous. But walk (or limp) I did.

I lived in Manhattan before cell phones had kicked in. Preoccupied people on the streets had to look up, acknowledge one another, find a way to maneuver the masses to stay on top of their game. In all the rushing, humanity still had a place for humanity.

I arrived at the photography lab. A tall, dark man was sitting at the front of a room. He wore glasses and was checking out all the beautiful women arriving to learn at his feet. A large group had gathered, a mixture of young hipsters, New York socialites, middle management types, and some truly weird individuals who befuddled us all. Ah, New York.

Almost immediately, a tall, brown woman was chatting with everyone. Her coolness was of the highest caliber, her clothes the most unique I had ever witnessed.

She seemed to have arrived with a tall, blond woman, a model I recognized from fashion magazines.

I was intimidated by their worldliness, beauty, and skinniness. They ate hamburgers for lunch and put too much sugar in their coffee. They took smoking breaks, while I ate cookies and read French medieval texts. Or just sat there. It was slippery outside.

The teacher gave us our first assignment.

We roamed around the neighborhood for two hours, attempting to discreetly photograph people, pigeons, building corners, shadows, and drifts of snow.

That tall, brown woman was so nice to me. She asked me questions and got me to laugh.

I wasn't sure how to read her at first. I have not had much experience with lesbian flirtations, if that was what she was doing, but I do know that I felt icky and flattered at the same time by someone actually paying attention to me, or at least acknowledging that I was in the room along with everyone else.

The teacher told us to shoot as much as possible until the following week, when we would be developing our photographs from start to finish.

I still have some of the photos today: the snowflakes delicately sprinkled on the corner edge of a 1950s Packard; the old lady sitting on a brick wall, her back turned toward me; Mrs. Rothschild's one hundred-year-old hands perched atop her piano keys; the plastic bag dangling from the tree outside my window.

When I returned to photography class the following week, the tall, dark woman was there. She had wrapped herself in a burlap robe. I was standing next to her as we developed our photos.

I asked her where she got her robe. She told me she had purchased it on her trip to Tibet, spoken as casually as if everyone has taken a trip to Tibet and purchased a robe.

She asked me, "Is your leg hurt?"

No, I countered. "I have an artificial leg."

She paused. Smiled. Stepped away.

"Now *that's* hot."

Another life changer had entered my world.

This is Courage Management Technology
Hey, I know you.
I've never found any opiate like the crutches of Christ.
But if I do, I'll let you know.
Eventually we all ask why, why, why?
Skeptic, meet your Maker.
He is standing right there to answer your call.

CHAPTER 22

I see spirals everywhere, turning in upon themselves.
They are the shapes of the universe,
intertwined DNA, fig leaves,
nautilus shells, fiddleheads, dogs chasing after their tails,
even the statues of Jesus on the cross,
with his loincloth coiled at his pelvis.

I am swathed in the garment of the universe,
an endless supply of spiraling galaxies
and magnetic attractions.
First I am in the center, then the edge,
clinging to the end of a long line of spirals,
gliding along a stream of stars, wrapping
my body like a possum around a sprig of pine branch,
or floating on the crystalline structure of a snowflake.

Almost three-quarters of me knows
this to be true. The other one-quarter wants
answers. Indefinitely.

I took it upon myself to meet with staff at the posttreatment follow-up program at the cancer clinic where I was treated. I hadn't been on the pediatric ward in years. The outpatient chemotherapy clinic, with its blue walls and high ceilings, was an attempt at cheerfulness.

It was a crowded place with a lot going on: social workers buzzing through, families consulting with nursing staff, doctors, fellow sufferers.

When I walked in, I went to the understaffed front desk. The ward clerk was handsome, a Hispanic man with a long, black ponytail. He was cute, but curt. My emotional padding deflated. I was left with a familiar tense knot in my throat. I waited, interminably, for my doctor to show up. Someone who could tell me what would happen. After an hour, I timidly approached the front desk again. I filled out a form, finally, while trying to hold back a rush of tears. It was no use. Uncontrollable sobs soaked through; the receptionist held my hand, as if he had finally woken up to the fact that he worked in a cancer center.

My sadness, fear, and anger mounted as I met with uptight volunteers, unfriendly social workers, and busy nurses (who gave me more forms to fill out, more instructions to "have a seat please," and brisk "we'll be with you shortly" dismissals).

Finally, after another two hours of waiting (Did I mention this program is voluntary? Yes, a part of their research on long-term cancer survivors), I met with a nurse who was part of the posttreatment program. She was well informed, but her agenda kept me from speaking about what I'd been through. She questioned my memory, basing everything on written charts from twenty years ago. Like so many other specialists, she was jaded, and apparently more of an expert than I.

After the empathy-lacking interview, the waiting continued—long and full of frightful imaginings, as desperately ill patients were wheeled in and out of rooms. One man caught my eye in the midst of this. He was devastatingly handsome, incredibly radiant, and quite disfigured. With one look we acknowledged our fortifying internal power, our flint-like determination, and the bittersweet comfort of sharing this awareness.

My day ended with the entrance of a tall Italian girl prancing through the unit. She seemed a recent graduate of the school of terminal illness. She knew where to go, what to do, but she was on the outskirts. Her sentence had been completed. Soft and radiant, her hair growing back in clumps, she seemed to exhale relief. "It's over and you didn't get me." I followed her trail past a long opening where people lay in hospital beds, receiving their treatments. A nurse standing near me said this row of beds continued all the way to the pediatric unit. It was a depressing view, all these sick people lined up in a row, faceless, hairless, and nameless to me. They were losing their identities. The Italian girl had found hers again.

So had I!

So had I!

Listen to the sound of butterfly wings
When you are alone on a mountaintop
Having climbed the summit so many times
You know the routine
You achieved the high
You overcame the odds
As usual no one was watching, not even you
You climbed that mountain thinking you had done it on your own
This time is different
This time you are the mistress of nothing, and the recipient of all that is good
To hear
Alone on a mountaintop
Is where you begin
To remember who you have always been
A child who can hear the wings of butterflies

Chapter 23

Hope is a pulse
It comes and goes with each moment of sanctification
That day his four friends carried the paralytic over the roof
And dropped him into a hole
Jesus was there

The longitudinal studies are in. Childhood cancer can be a catastrophe in your adult life.

It's not so much the massive side effects that can creep up along the way, which are many. It's the story of what it means to be a death defier in a world where death, and the business of escaping death, is "not something we talk about." Most people want to hear about the victory.

What does a girl do with all the pent-up knowledge she has learned along the way? She is bursting with words she does not know how to speak. Will they listen? Can they?

There is only one solution for her: she must dance.

One day when I didn't know what to do with my life, I found a picture of a man in a wellness center catalog. He was smiling, his head turned to the side, his arms open wide.

He was teaching a training that combined yoga and dance.

I heard the butterfly wings amidst the storm of dialysis. There was no hesitation. All was clear.

It is like that when you hear butterfly wings.

I signed up immediately.

It was early summer when I arrived at the training.

My bag was heavy, as was my worry. Would people stare at me? How far away was the dialysis center? Would I get good medical treatment? Was there handicapped parking? What would I eat at this vegetarian sanctuary, with my low sodium, low potassium, and low phosphorous dialysis diet? How would I deal with all that sweat when I was limited to four cups of fluid per day? Would I be okay? Would people like me? Would I be able to get back into the building late at night after my dialysis treatment? Would my leg survive all the dancing? Would I be okay? Would I be okay?

I was directed to my dormitory, where I met women from all over the world, excited to begin dance training the next day. I unpacked and took a walk through the facility.

My first shock was the bookstore. My awe of this place as a spiritual center was quickly diminished. How could "they" be so materialistic! It took me a day to get over that narrow sentiment, when I saw all the cute yoga clothes lining the back wall.

I strolled past the large bulletin board next to registration. I salivated at the offerings the center provided. Workshops, yoga classes, hikes, wellness lectures, massage. This place was for seekers, like me.

Upstairs on the second floor was the cafeteria. The menu made it clear. I would be very hungry during my training. I would eat salad. And bread. And even then, how much fluid was in each lettuce leaf? How would I get any protein when legumes were prohibited? How much cooked eggplant and zucchini could I have? Kale, don't even try. Would the tofu destroy my bones or give me a heart attack? Every bite could be my last bite.

The atmosphere was relaxed, set in the mountains overlooking a lake, but I would remain on my tiptoes while I was there, never quite touching the mountain grass. Dialysis made me stand on the perimeter of life. There was always a chance the mountains could be taken away from me forever. Until I began to dance again, I lived my life at a distance from reality. Hope entangled me, smothering me with its obligation for me to have faith, yet hope kept me alive.

It takes a lot of fuel to fire up hope when hope is your only means of survival.

That first night our group met on the second floor in a former chapel. St. Francis was there at the altar, holding a bird in his hand.

Good. Not too weird. Yet.

The place smelled like damp carpet.

"This ain't no Canyon Ranch," I mused silently.

We introduced ourselves through movement, one person after another.

Then the dance began.

My walls crumbled quickly.

By the end of the evening, my feet were almost on the ground.

I have never been so turned on in my entire life.

I had finally been rooted by my dance.

Historian

Some people need to see the buildings
with their gunshot wounds and crumbling towers
Some people need to read books by experts

I get my history from

Stomping feet
Slithering fingers
Chest presses
Three-foot leaps in the air
Deep squats
Gyrating hips
Tiptoes through tall grasses
Hands behind ears
Shimmying shoulders
Flat palms
Undulating spines
Chopping elbows
Pounding hearts
Flying trapezoids
Upturned chins
Smug faces
Joyous eyes
Hopeful shouts
Rhythm

I get my history from the rhythms of the people.

CHAPTER 24

I get another email.
Or, I receive a phone call
Or, someone looks at me . . . just wrong.
Or, my heart is terrified.
Or, my head is hooked onto
the same scene from twelve years ago.
Or, I compare myself to someone
else and it hurts.
Or, I haven't finished something important
that I have wanted to finish.
Or, I didn't speak up when I should have.
Or, I should be much further
ahead in my life.
Or, I should know by now what to do.
Or, I'm not trying hard enough.
Or, I'm not connected anymore.
Or, I have a dream.
Or, I am misunderstood in conversation.
Or, I'm tired.

Or . . .

I want answers.
When I spiral.
Here is what He showed me.

There is a tall, wide oak tree in a large field.
The tree has been there for hundreds of years.
I see some leaves fall to the ground.
A chronicle of resentments,
dropping so lightly to blanket the earth.
No, that's not it. That is not enough.
I am not the let-it-go-and-it-will-be-all-right kind of girl.

I want something of substance.

I see the acorns budding on the branches.
Acorns: compressed forms of matter, spirals of hope,
seed, life force, and dignity, not
a cloud of resentment to be found.
They are all innocent. Some will grow into trees.
Some trees will have diseases.
Some trees will be maimed
by the weather, time, people.
Some trees will be cut down.
Some trees will die of old age.
They are all innocent.

This is what it is like for me when I move to a new place. I scramble around, seeking places I can call home, like yoga studios, coffee shops, nature paths, and churches.

I take long drives in my car to capture the landscape of the people. More than anything, the people matter.

I wonder if I'll ever belong or choose to never belong, being myself unequivocally.

That first Sunday after I moved unexpectedly—after a breakup, after leaving my home north of Boston, after selling everything, after my insurance was denied in another state due to my "pre-existing condition"—my body still riddled with shock, I was determined to go to church.

I happened upon the Episcopalians.

I had moved so quickly, an urgent flip from my original plans, setting me reeling into extreme action. I dragged heavy boxes of clothes and computer equipment over sheets of ice to my new makeshift space. I hadn't had the strength to open them all, so I was left with a peacock feather-print dress and my black fishnet stockings.

I smiled as I entered the church. Their eyes grasped this new face of mine, then quickly found their way to my hosiery.

In those moments, I often choose to lift my skirt just a little higher.

Oh Beauty Seeker
She is getting a message
From someone
The despised part that is touching
her face with a washcloth
Has gone far away again
There is repulsion
Like when she tries to eat those peas
Or touch the messy meal with her fingers

It is upsetting

She endures it over and over
In different settings
In different ways

And the music plays in the background
So far away

No one is there, really

Only one of them gets to be beautiful

And we know who that is

CHAPTER 25

I have written lists upon lists
of what I want in a man,
recorded on pages of paper,
in journals, and on random walks near oceans.
Every requirement has been met . . . just not all in one package.

A carpenter, like Jesus, who had
an air of sophistication √
A man who had lived in a specific region of Italy √
A man with an interesting ring √
A man who twiddled with my fingers just so √
A cute Jersey boy who played soccer √
An owner of a private jet √
A former hockey player √
A cigar smoker √
An Italian √
A man with an accent √
A piano player √
A lover with as much stamina as I have √
A race car driver √
A man who had a pilot's license √
A crisply dressed man √
A charmer √
A risk taker √
An architect √
A photographer √
A gentleman cowboy with an
Ivy League education √
A man with a past √
A man with large hands √

I will give you the desires of your heart, says He.

Well?

B, my first real love, found me absolutely gorgeous, which meant, of course, that he loved me.

P thought I was captivating. He held my hand and mauled me with his French/Swiss kisses. That was LA.

Then there was M, the adopted Mexican; and S, the Texan getting his masters at the Kennedy School of Government; the weird British guy from a store in Cambridge; and ST, a French chef—they got me through my year at Harvard. My boobs were finally touched. The Brit thought I was the most sexually experienced woman he had ever met. Ha! I was still a virgin. ST wanted to marry me for his green card. Couldn't he at least take me out dancing first?

Still wanting to be "equally yoked with a Christian man" (until I got to New York and actually met some of them), it never dawned on me that dangerous dressing might send off a certain vibe. I just wanted to be desirable, in spite of . . .

In spite of . . .

In spite of the visible wounds so conspicuously hidden . . . or something like that.

I'm guessing prepubescence was still in effect.

AR met me on the steps of the Metropolitan in Manhattan. I wore a tightly fitted, Lycra, above-the-knee, flower-print dress—the same killer outfit I wore the day I obtained my French student visa. AR, my Latvian Gregory Peck, opened his thick, muscular, working-class arms, and his smile, as I walked up the stairs toward him, then ignored him completely. He turned his head to look at me as I shyly entered the museum, where I prowled the corridors, hoping that I'd be noticed for my bod, not my artificial leg, which was being debuted that day. I took the elevator to the top deck to view the Henry Miller sculptures. I was so nervous, then angry with myself for not at least acknowledging him—but that was all part of my adolescent game. When I left the museum, he was still on the steps, waiting. I ignored him again. Geez! He followed me down Fifth Avenue. His first awkward words to me were, "It is hard?" We went to Bergdorf's for coffee. "Ahh, an angel from heaven has come to me," he anxiously uttered. No more virginity! My father wanted to buy him a flower shop.

"Congratulations. It is finished." Didn't Jesus say that somewhere?

Before I left for Paris, he kissed me at the corner of two avenues in downtown Manhattan. A dreamy scene in my eyes, until I moved to Paris, saw *Taxi Driver*, and worried that my Latvian friend could have been a replica.

He sent me a card. "When man is not ready he cannot be lover, but woman's emptiness is always waiting."

I told people—Penny at the English institute, an Italian stranger on the train to Toulon, Sophie's friends—I was "in love." But it felt strange in my throat when I said it.

ST's mother took me to his apartment in the 18th in Paris. We faxed him in the Caribbean, where he worked. She kept pursuing me all year, taking me on meat tours and out to drab cafés with sticky cups. Hoping I'd become her daughter-in-law. But ST, I am guessing, had another American in mind—one from the islands.

ST's friend from the streets was in a family business, Au Lapin Agile. I thought for sure my cute, tight outfit would get a few dates out of him. He taught me how to swear in French without using words.

I met AA when I was taking my daily walk through the 5th. He was doodling architecture on a scrap of paper. That weekend we walked along a part of the Seine that nobody goes to. We crashed some art openings on the Left Bank. He told me he wanted to be known for doing something frivolous in life. He was so pretty, as Madame Gely commented. She couldn't get enough of him. I couldn't get enough of him. He could get enough of me. Three years later, when I went to San Francisco, I would find him in the crowd during Halloween's Gay Parade in the Castro. I turned around. There he was. That frightened him immensely.

Church boys were a special breed altogether. They were cold and yet sort of warm; maybe because they loved God but wanted to jump my bones, too? I thought every one of them would be my husband.

When I moved to NYC, there was a whole new lot of bachelors to conquer.

D was walking by my building on 84th and York. He had a Chow Chow. He was studying Shakespeare. He took my hand and recited Romeo and Juliet's balcony scene. We went to the dog park. His dog was aggressive. He blamed everyone else. We had lots of fun on rooftops and in banks.

My mother set me up with a man who told me I had excellent bone structure, which would be good for our children. Lucky for me, I couldn't have children.

G and E had double lives, but I was too naïve to know it. They loved being with me, in bookstores, coffee shops, walks through the park. At least E was Irish and Jewish. That was something.

PA made the pizzas at my fave restaurant on the Upper East Side. He would come to my table to ask if I needed more water. We walked around the reservoir. He did sit-ups on the park bench. We attended Brazilian church together. We made out in the Egyptian section of the Met. He said, "It is hard," with a glaring look of passion, like a tiger in heat. I had NO IDEA what he meant.

PI saved me from the angst of beginning dialysis. He played Spanish guitar until two in the morning, then slithered up next to me for hours of double Scorpio pleasure.

The dryness began in Massachusetts. What is it with those men? Are they too chilly to notice a woman? Don't know how to flirt? Did I lose my cute gene? How is it women actually snag a man in this state? I couldn't seem to do it.

J fell in love with me immediately. It happened the day I stayed in Lake Placid to recover from dialysis, when I finally decided to stop looking. I went to the fancy coffee shop. He came right toward me, chatted me up. He was *so* cute. Big blue eyes, muscles everywhere. Charm, charm, charm. I married him. My weekends alone started soon afterwards. The sexless honeymoon turned into the sexless marriage. He loved something more and I couldn't compete with fermented brews of grain that turned themselves into Vodka. I always dreamed of the other woman when he was on a binge. Was she real, or was she alcohol? It ended.

R told me he loved me in sign language within a month. He moved in with me. After three years he moved out. He didn't call.

I tried online dating.

After many months I was exhausted with the endless emails, phone calls, dates, and learning to say no graciously.

There *were* a few gifts.

I had hours of pleasure with a thirty-year-old Greek and a few boys in their twenties.

I needed to relive my lost ages.

My ex-husband was gorgeous—Steve McQueen.
My ex-husband was charming—Cary Grant.
My ex-husband was sexy rough—Tommy Lee Jones.
My ex-husband was a Marlboro man—Sam Elliott.
My ex-husband was funny—Jim Carrey.
My ex-husband was a rough-around-
the-edges Jersey boy—Bruce Springsteen.
My ex-husband was a little in your face—Ray Liotta.
My ex-husband was a deep m-f'er—John Lennon.
My ex-husband knew how to get out of any trouble—James Bond.
My ex-husband was street smart—Quincy Jones.
My ex-husband wore his heart
on his sleeve—Sam Shepard.
My ex-husband spoke when
he had something real to say—Clint Eastwood.
My ex-husband cleaned up well—Johnny Depp.
My ex-husband was a phenomenally
talented chef—Bobby Flay.
My ex-husband was an
incredible designer—Frank Lloyd Wright.
My ex-husband was very connected
to nature—Any hunky guy from Alaska.
My ex-husband was physically strong—Arnold S.
My ex-husband was an alcoholic—my grandfather.

We were at the Cascade Lakes I told him I was on dialysis.
He turned to me, stating in his
Jersey accent, "You'll be alright, kid."
We were engaged a week later.

After the wedding, I got scared.

The endless nights alone, the
conversation flipping to make
it seem like I was losing my mind.
The lack of sex. The violent verbal outbursts.
The calls from police stations, jails,
different states. The lack of calls or
any communication whatsoever.
The dramatic apologies. The no-shows

after major surgeries and blood
pressure drops. The complete lack
of remorse. The constant criticism
for the smallest infraction.

The ears fine-tuned to detect
the turn of the kitchen doorknob.
Would he come home? And if so,
which him would he be?
The uncelebrated anniversaries.
The imposed silence. The sequestering
away from family and friends because
"our love was so much more real
than anyone else's could ever be."
The wasted hours at courthouses.
The wasted money. The bailouts
after countless quit jobs and firings.
The lengthy cover-up it took to appear
happy to the not-so-deceived family.

The terrible digestive problems
from too much stuffing of words and feelings.
The constant sense of danger for lack
of personal safety. The guilt
of wanting him to leave me.
The terror of being alone through
all this dialysis (though technically I was anyway).
The thousands of pages of journal writing
dedicated to the possibility of hope
and the reality of desperation.

Chapter 26

I am not afraid of love.
I tap my palms.
They aren't Jesus, so I shouldn't complain.

I just want to be loved.
I am, and I can't take it in.
If I did, what would happen to me?

I would see too much beauty.
I would have to see this stump as beautiful.
I would have to be visible.

I could die from the exposure.

I know how to die—I have done it so many times.

That is the mind speaking. Run for cover.

I have always . . .

Risen above.

High on my things-I-would-like-to-try-but-haven't list was entering a Mrs. America pageant.

There is not one ounce of Mrs. America blood in me.

I prefer most things Western European: the food (except England and Germany, of course), the clothing, the people, the men, the china, the topography, the culture, the history, the many languages, and the pace. I draw the line at the bathrooms, showers, and medical facilities. I am mixed about those.

I was surprised by how easy it was to be accepted into the Mrs. Massachusetts pageant. Basically, I needed to fill out an application and pay some serious money.

My husband was very upset by my desire to go through with the pageant.

"Why do you need someone out there to tell you how beautiful you are?"

At the time I bought his argument. Now I wonder why he was so opposed. Well, actually, I don't wonder. He is no longer a part of my life. However, the picture of me walking across the stage in my red Chinese dress that won Best Evening Gown is somewhere in storage. I have proof (in addition to my scars) that I've participated in things that have made me afraid.

I drove to the pageant by myself, since my husband refused to join me. As I came up the driveway I saw a flurry of beauty queens in tight, short skirts, with perfect coifs, skinny bodies, translucent skin shimmering with glitter, smiles that were glued into place, and entourages surrounding them. Then there was me. Little, natural me.

I realized immediately that I'd come ill-equipped for the proceedings. All I brought was a tiny bag filled with minimal makeup, my heel leg, my one-piece black bathing suit and black wrap, a little hair spray, a suit for the "interview," and my red dress.

I smiled warmly at everyone I met. At least my nails were done. But my Audrey Hepburn hair was far too short. I could see by the falling locks of hair that I was outmaneuvered. I sat down midrow, next to a few sort-of-nice ladies. There was no open hostility, just a general discomfort at my presence. *Wait until they see me in my bathing suit!*

Eventually, the proceedings began. Everyone talked in half voices, a sort of quasi-honesty tinged with forced sincerity and a dash of encouragement.

After all, there was nothing about this contest based on merit. It was genetics, plus a bit of working out and a wealth of knowledge about makeup application that would allow a Mrs. to win.

The staff prepared us for what to expect. I got nervous when they told us we would be removing our wrap during bathing suit time, and even more nervous because I was first up in that category. Not that there was so much competition: seven girls to compete for the Mrs. Massachusetts title. They all set up their trunks in the room out back. These girls were professional!

I got dressed in the bathroom.

The first leg of the pageant began with the interviews. We went around a circle of "experts" who asked questions about our platform. Platform? What platform? I was so unprepared.

By the umpteenth person going in front of me responding to the question, "Who is a great role model for you?" and having *every* woman respond, "Mrs. George W.," I couldn't wait to answer.

I came up to the last interviewer, a tightwad with a face of steel.

"Whom do you admire?"

"The Dalai Lama." Which led her to ask, "Do you think your PhD candidacy will hinder you from adequately representing Mrs. Massachusetts?" *Ooh, a trick question; egad! How should I respond?*

The luncheon came next. Salad and some sort of protein. And, ooh, shouldn't we all indulge in that chocolate? Tee hee hee. I couldn't wait until I got up on stage with my bathing suit—all ninety-eight pounds of me!

The crowds started to gather around 2:30 p.m. My two friends, with graying hair and unshaven armpits, both healers wearing earth goddess clothing (textured organic cotton in muted mauve and sage green), sat in the audience cheering me on. Next up was evening gowns. I worked it, because unlike all the other women who wore gowns of extravagant prices, I got mine online for less than one hundred dollars. My sexy smile came as a result of my shopping coup.

Then came bathing suits. I walked boldly onto the stage in my glam, forties-style, black, ruched bathing suit, which enhanced the few curves I had beneath my beautiful black wrap, accentuated by my prosthetic leg displaying my clunky, forties-style, thick-soled heels. Another shopping coup smile emerged. I took a breath and cupped my elbows behind my back, ashamed by the visibility of needle marks along my punctured arms. First there was silence, then clapping and whistling, then . . . assumably horror, for many began looking away.

It was time for me to bring out the Scorpio eyes.

I stood there confidently as the interviewer interrogated me about my platform. So I made something up; something like, "I will be an example to women young and old in Massachusetts that all things are possible, that beauty of the soul is as important, if not more so, than exterior beauty." I know my friends clapped, but just about everyone else in the audience was silent.

And the competitors, while plausibly horrified and moved and inspired, were *still* noticeably jealous. Part of me wanted to protest, "Oh yeah ladies, let's see how confident you'd be if *you* were missing your leg, or had all these scars. What would it take you to feel beautiful?"

Damn, maybe I am pretty after all. Or, real beauty takes guts.

Needless to say, my story was not enough to win the contest. I came in sixth. I felt dizzy from the visibility. But, hey, I was still smiling, utterly proud of my accomplishment. I had entered a Mrs. Pageant, gave it my best effort, and I was alive—dialyzed, cancered, amputated, scar-ridden body and all. The other girl, the one who thought for sure she would win, as her gown was *so* costly, her bod *so* delish, her insistence on her sincerity *so* close to convincing, came in fifth. Her disappointment was *so* obvious.

I had not a disappointed bone in my body for the event.

Years later I would be sitting on the floor, meditating on the map of my trauma-scarred body, reflecting some aspect of the universal body, experiencing a kind of beautiful compassion. I put a dash of compassion there. Now over here. Oh and here, a place I had forgotten. Who knew I could radiate even more? I am finding the beauty. Over and over I am finding it.

Step out
into beauty

It takes that much
To make the first step
Into clouds and rivers

It takes that much
Just to see it as it is
Face to face

Put a name to it
See it
Touch it

Taste it
And when you feel
The soft blanket of grass beneath
Or hear the swollen sound
You've arrived

Perhaps a new place
Or the same place
Only different I should know
I passed by beauty many times
Until one day it stopped me,

Before I had time to run
She told me to see her fully
I couldn't help but look
I was so intrigued by her calm demeanor
I dove in full force.

She took me to the deepest corners
The darkest places
Her response was always the same
"Do you see how beautiful you are?
Can't you just taste it?"

And I did.

The taste was familiar and not entirely forgotten
It was my reminder—
With you I am well pleased
She said peace covered me like a blanket
I never had to run away again.

Chapter 27

If I accept this body, it means
I have to accept my humanity.
I am torn between heaven and earth.
The leg is cut off.
I am not completely here, am I?
How can one woman
have so many body stories
and yet be so halfheartedly
interested in living in this body.

It is so hard to live in this body,
I told God.
Holy Spirit replied, "Yes, but
I love living in this body."
Marsha replied, "Good,
then you figure it out."

"Why not trust ourselves less and God more?" read the sign on Route 41 in the Berkshires. I was rushing to get to the last weekend of my movement therapy training, the conclusion of nearly one year of intense study. I was late, having decided to take the back roads from Boston on through. I needed time to drive, see the mountains, feel my feelings, and prepare to be in a group setting. It was the same old story, feeling like I didn't belong in the group, then wanting to belong and not wanting to belong all at the same time.

I was feeling okay. After all, I had a new kidney. I was divorced. No longer did I need to call home to make sure my husband was sober or actually working at his job. The drive in the country gave me time. I wanted time to reflect on the past year and all I had gained.

Then that sign appeared.

I suppose for most people of faith the message of the sign would bring them comfort. You know:"Let go and let God," "Just surrender into trust," "God is always with us," "Just trust God," "God's got your back."

Not so with me! Anger, frustration, disgust, and pure sadness rushed through me, seeping into my bones moments before I was to arrive at the training. Suddenly, all my thoughts, my observations, my preparedness for the weekend seemed distant pulses, slight glimpses into a now-foggy year. All that was left was raw emotion.

I pulled over, one street before the building that was hosting my training. I would be really late.

I had to feel whatever this was.

It was so annoying, all this crying, my makeup dripping down my face. My increasingly red eyes and my heaving chest had a mind of their own. Funny how I never made the connection that day to the fact that I was studying how to unleash trapped emotions in the body in order to heal hidden pain. That was for *other* people, not me.

Normally I had the power to clean myself up and brave on through. Upsetting experiences were another day at the office for me. "What else is new?" had been my mantra for years.

It wasn't so much the "trusting God more"part of the sign that upset me, at least at first. It was the "trusting ourselves less"part of the message that infuriated me.

I had spent the last twenty years learning how to trust my body again after spending years in the blame and shame camp.

Why in the world would I want to trust myself less, for God's sake?

Who was this pastor who came up with this silly message anyway?

The truth is, with all this damn inner work I was doing, the more I trusted myself and my BODY, the more connected I felt with God. If I trusted myself less and God more, I'd be back where I started, now wouldn't I? Afraid that God was going to stick it to me again was in no way going to make me trust life again, ever.

There is a reason I was meant to feel God in my body. All these scars, my half limb, my cell sadness, these are body stories that need reckoning, not derision. My scars need to be trusted. So do my memories.

God is found in my scars. I can trust my scars. They are real, reminders that God and I got through the pain together. Why shortchange my Maker?

There are so many cuts.
Some are deep. Some are shallow. All were painful.

Chapter 28

There was a moment when
I lost my way
I could have trail blazed
Chopped through
After all, I bring myself wherever I go
This was no answer
Secret energies to overcome
Were just fired up nerves enraging the system
I decided to stay
Believing, for once, that this tree
Had never been struck down
But was standing strong
Fully fortified
Let angels come to rest their wings on my branches

My life is a series of cuts. This is a dream.

Biopsy cut—the first cut. Ever. Four inches long. On the outside of my left ankle. A little girl walks by with a limp in her left ankle. She's cute. So was I. Really cute. I wake up. I am nauseous. I have never thrown up like this before. Welcome to your new life. You'll get it after a while.

I'm cold in this hospital room, alone. The lights, the large beds, the separate accommodations, kids I've never met before.

Welcome to your new routine. Those kids will go home. You will stay.

Please don't leave me alone here. I am very scared.

No one reads me a story. No one tucks me in. I don't have any friends.

I run away.

I get in trouble.

"You're not scared"

'No you're not."

"Okay."

'You're mad."

"Okay."

I eat Jesus so now I am all better. I'll show them.

But it is never the same, ever. Lost in a world of permanent separation.

No hand-holding for you darling.

I . . . don't . . . know . . . how . . . to . . . do . . . this.

Thrown into first grade halfway through the year, I don't know any of the kids. I can't keep up. I am so behind. I go visit my mother, who teaches second grade. She is very angry that I bothered her.

I run away in second grade, more than once. More than twice. Suddenly everyone is concerned.

Saturdays are for Daddy. He hugs me lots and gives me presents, but he won't let me cry much.

I find a new crowd in grade school. The fringe group, the out skirters. They are cool, too. But they are very sadistic. I thought I was bad. They get away with it. They grow up popular. I have a few friends.

I . . . don't know . . . how . . . to . . . do . . . this.

Lump returns. The second cut. Biopsy.

There goes the leg. Wipe out. Third cut—very deep. I was allowed to cry and "feel sorry for myself." How about FEEL period?! The fourth cut.

Thrown into Sloan Kettering. Why am I going up that elevator by myself, at thirteen, to CHEMOTHERAPY? Are you kidding me? I don't know any better. All those hovering parents. I get to make my own rules by lying.

The girls in high school think I am snobby.

I am separate. I really only like one girl. She is still my friend, forty years later. The others weren't worth it, as I suspected.

The bladder bleeds. Over and over. They stick the cauterizing iron inside the urethra. Fifth cut.

Sixth cut. Seventh cut. They'll get it right. My bladder will be all right.

Arms have been mutilated again and again, Burned. Scar tissue. Veins in the back of the hands have permanently thrombosed. Does a poke count as a cut? If so, I am up to at least five thousand cuts by now. None of these cuts are self-inflicted.

Hair goes. Cut number eight.

College. I refind Jesus. Hope renewed. Bladder dies. They open up the belly and place a urostomy bag on the right side. Cut number nine, ten, and eleven. Constant inner worry comes about this urostomy. Who will ever go out with me? Cut number twelve.

I love being a Christian. I don't like the Christians. I barely tell them my story. They wouldn't really understand. They are so much more spiritual than I.

But something really isn't right with them. Really.

Some years of silence follow, a respite from the physical suffering. I really don't know how to relate to the world. I move to LA and try my hand at a design business. I am terrible at it. I never have a real boyfriend. I learn about beauty and insecurity, I never felt so bad about myself before, or good when girls looked at me with jealousy. It was so confusing. Guys barely noticed me. Cut number thirteen.

My business is a complete wash. I am too shy about selling my stuff. I feel so unworthy, otherwise I would have two legs, a bladder, and a boyfriend. I am no good at thinking I am good at anything. I have no excitement about selling. I hate it. It shows. But I love the line I create.

I get a new prosthesis. I can't walk in it. I am in pain all the time. Girls I know all have boyfriends. I have friends, sort of, I am too bound up, but people tell me I am so cool. I sit my true friends down to tell them I had cancer and an artificial leg. They are all moved. It is the first time. I say the words coolly, "I had cancer and I lost my left leg." I am not there when I say the words.

I go in for a checkup. There could be a problem, they forget I am in the waiting room. For six hours I wait. I hate doctors. I decided they are my enemies. It is the only way.

My sister marries a doctor. At first I am afraid to accept him as a human being. He is so kind.

A routine checkup reveals extremely high blood pressure. My blood pressure is too high. My kidneys are not well. I am sad but not that concerned. The girl in the waiting room has kidney disease. She frightens me. Cut number fourteen.

When I return to the East Coast I am in graduate school over and over. At Harvard I can't tell the story. They are too smart, too intellectual, too agnostic. They won't care. I'll be smart and tough like them, I'll be high achieving and dismissive of feelings.

I am consumed with sadness, but I don't know it. I am so lonely, but I figure it is because I am in graduate school. The pretty dancer talks to me in a dismissive way. I think maybe it must be me. I try to pretend to like her and be her friend, because she is so articulate, well-liked, and fun. But I am jealous and she sees through me. I waste my entire year at Harvard worrying about this woman in my spare time. I awaken sexuality, but only slightly. Too many scars. The church is a safe haven for denying me the truth of my body. I tell my dates the fantasy: the overcoming. They will not see my scars or my urostomy. I cover that up with master finesse.

Paris is lonely, but beautiful. Which is better? Beauty or friendship?

What do I call myself?

My New York PhD. That would be an achievement.

I have a hard time getting around New York. I can't take taxis all the time as they are too expensive.

I attend a cool church with lots of single, good-looking men. I start dating. I have such pretty hair. I don't eat enough. But I am thin and pretty and men are noticing. After LA this is good news. It is all still a fantasy. Who would really stay if they knew about the scars?

I don't know how to tell the truth about my body.

They rewire my urinary system. Biopsy—cut number fourteen and a half. Belly cut deep down the middle. Cut number fourteen and three-quarters. Inner belly is cut and bladder is cut from my body. Cut number fourteen and seven-eighths.

I still can't believe I made it through cancer. I tell everybody in Bible study. They think I am great. I am known for my story. But no one really knows me.

My roommate is very popular and pretty. Her prayers are always answered. The doctor tells me my kidneys are failing. My roommate doesn't want to be around my old, inexpressible negativity. I go to a Christian therapist who is not very wise. I know more than she does. I edit what I say because I feel she will judge me; I am at the cusp of accepting now that these Christians might not know everything.

I am confirmed when I tell people my kidneys are failing. Their responses are so trite and pithy. No one holds my hand and lets me cry. No one. Job's friends sat with him for seven days without a word. I must be selfish for even bringing up my kidneys and not bringing my fears to God. I AM bringing them to God. Only He can't hold my hand.

I go back to Catholicism. The church is fancy; the music is spectacular. This is authentic.

Oh, did I mention the numerous pneumonias I have had when I went away to foreign countries, or the countless blisters on my leg that kept me from amazing sightseeing? I have learned to adapt and accept. I ask for very little and appreciate all.

It sure would be nice to freely go where I want to go, completely unencumbered.

This is why heaven seems awfully enticing sometimes.

When the kidneys fail, the doctors put a catheter in my neck. They scrape and cut my throat to get the tube down into my heart. Cut number fifteen. Cut number sixteen is in New York on the left arm. A long incision is made to place the GORE-TEX graft on the surface, yet another scar to hide.

I am hiding my left leg, my stomach, and now my left arm. A few years later the right lower arm follows, riddled with cuts from hundreds of needles. There are four or five more catheters in the neck. Cuts sixteen, seventeen, eighteen, ninety, twenty.

Weekends are lost to recovering from dangerous infections due to the catheters piercing my heart. This is very frightening and so much to manage. Another weekend or week or month is lost. Cut number twenty-one.

It is possible to have a life on dialysis, but there is so much to control. Day in and day out I had to be brave. Dialysis is threatening with potential heart attacks, significant loss of freedom (cut number twenty-two), diabetes, neuropathy, vision trouble, bone loss, amputations of fingers and toes, mental incapacitation. It was a lot to see, every other day, year in and year out. Cut number twenty-three.

I couldn't get out of dialysis if I wanted to stay alive. I watched other people my age build careers, homes, families, fulfill dreams, while I attempted to recover yet again from another treatment, perhaps watch a movie. Cut number twenty-four.

My life is sacred.

I deal with dialysis staff so I can feel safe. My life is in their hands every other day. Cut number twenty-five.

Why in the world would I want to stay? Who knows?

I begin my yoga path. I was. Meant to be. Staying.

They prepare me for a new kidney.

I aggressively poke my old makeshift bladder to prepare for my kidney. I am in the bathroom for hours. I need this bladder to work, but it doesn't. I collapse on the floor. Cut number twenty-six.

My middle must be cut again. There are deep cuts inside my belly, with more ilium cut, more left side cut, and more time cut. Cut number twenty-seven. The surgery wipes me out, but it is hopeful because new birth is coming.

Kidney comes four months later. Cut down the middle is deep and easy, but surgery is complicated. Cut number twenty-eight.

I leave my husband three weeks later. Cut number twenty-nine.

All is good.

I am alone again. I don't like this. Am I going to be single for the rest of my life? I want someone to hold my hand through all of this.

The weekends are dusty. Cut number thirty.

My hair is thin again. Cut number thirty-one. I am so disappointed. My heart is breaking. Funny what does it, isn't it?

The veins start to bulge on my back and right arm. I can't breathe or move or walk upstairs. I worry all the time, which is not good for my kidney. My soul hurts. My face gets swollen, the veins popping out on my face.

I don't want anymore Lord! I don't want any more. Not another self-image issue, please. Cut number thirty-two.

After almost a year with no answer, the physicians finally figure out what is wrong. Cut number thirty-three. They tell me I have congestive heart failure and "not to worry."Cut number thirty-four.

Okay.

Cut number thirty-five is the huge syringe poked through my ribs into my lung. Sure, I'll sign your consent form, just in case of a collapsed lung, infection, or that sort of thing. I wanted to breathe again.

The fluid in my abdomen is drawn out by a large syringe. Cut number thirty-six.

A biopsy on the kidney *(please not the kidney)* reveals nothing. Cut number thirty-seven.

The creatinine is very high, a precursor to kidney failure. Cut number thirty-eight.

The blood pressure is very high, a precursor to kidney failure. Cut number thirty-nine.

They want to open my groin as I drink sulfur that has "side effects."

Fear galore. Cut number forty.

They cancel the surgery. Cut number thirty-nine.

I drink the radioactive material with potential side effects (kidney failure) for another scan or two. Cuts forty and forty-one.

They decide to tie off the fistula (my dialysis access). A welcome cut number forty-two.

My blood pressure goes all over the place. My parents divorce. Cuts forty-three and forty-four.

My sweetheart looks in my eyes with more love than I ever thought possible. I finally have someone to hold my hand. Our hearts pulse together all the time. He is the prayer answered. I am never alone anymore. My heart is open. Cut number forty-five.

He leaves me for another woman.

Cut number forty-six.

I see that I am of great value.

Cut number forty-seven.

There will be more cuts.

I am worried.

God comes in the night to pierce my body with His love. Cuts are healing, slowly.

One day, I saw a worry.
I saw how its fetal shape deflated in the face of hope,
retreated into the cavern of fear,
turned its back on personal dreams,
separated itself from its form to keep from feeling any pain.

I saw this worry suspended in a place of no rest
using all its effort to stay hidden
from the faith over haulers and positive thinkers.
It had no hands or feet.

Unable to swim,
it was forced into a kind of contracted exile,
waiting for someone to fill it up,
not knowing if it would ever get the chance.
A second worry.

I lay the worry down in the dedicated crib as He had suggested.
His mother looked inside the worry with her love.
We waited, until the transaction was complete.

Filled with sweetness yet again,
I walked away unscathed,
just as Christ had promised.

There are millions of anonymous
mountain ranges around the globe.
He knows the name of every one of them.

CHAPTER 29

Let us see eye to eye
Tail to tail
Tongue to tongue
Wrapped in each other
The veil is lifted
We are left alone
Wild in the jungle
Free

I dreamed I met a black panther while I was walking alone on a dusty road. He emerged out of nowhere. Suddenly, three women appeared. They warned me that a black panther was standing in front of me. They huddled around me, appearing to protect me, but their eyes told a different story. They wanted me to stay afraid.

But I was already lying with the black panther, hugging him. I could feel his breath on me. His purr shook my body. I rubbed my fingers through his coarse fur. We had known each other since the beginning of time. The women disappeared. My panther and I remained.

The next day, when I woke up, I went for a mammogram, a test I had avoided for almost fifteen years. Why would I of all people want to know if I had cancer? I would never go through chemotherapy again. I would never let anything else get cut off again.

I did, however, have an incentive. My doctor wouldn't renew my long-standing prescription if I didn't go. Nothing like a little medical blackmail with good intentions to get a girl into a mammogram clinic.

The moment came. Breasts squished almost to oblivion. The nurse distracting me with gynecological jokes. She was an Italian mama kneading my breasts like a pound of ground beef. The ice-cold glass shelf tilted to an angle for the best view, the edge of the rounded glass shelf sticking its freezing metal frame into my awkwardly twisted neck.

The test was easy.

As usual, the waiting was not.

For days I hugged my black panther. He was licking my face when the doctor's call came.

He walked by my side as I endured a potential diagnosis, a barbaric biopsy (a word I haven't heard for many years), and more waiting.

Everyone had warned me about the surgeon. They said she was cold and unfriendly.

I loved her. She wore five-inch heels. She told me where she bought her outfits. She hugged me as I left her office. She hugged me after the biopsy. She hugged me when she told me the good news.

She, like the black panther, was my new ticket to fearlessness.

Cancer never leaves you.

But neither does your wild soul.

That eleventh year of dialysis, when
I could barely string onto hope, this happened.

God slammed the door in my face,
which broke my nose. I was determined
to get through that door. I had a few questions to ask that guy.
I looked at this big black door
of NO in front of me, laughed,
and kept on banging. I banged
and banged. I banged until
my knuckles were raw and bleeding.
I kept banging, because HE
had made a promise. "Knock
and the door shall be opened to you."
I believe God's promises.
After all, He is God.
I banged so hard on that big black
door of NO that my skin tore
to the bone and my fingers began to break.
I sobbed and sobbed from
the pain and the frustration.
I lifted my hand to look at it.
It was covered in blood.
The blood began to thicken and dry,
as I murmured, "Why, Why, why won't
you hear me, oh God. Why don't
you love me anymore?"
The weight of the loss of God's love
Dried my bones
Sagged my skin
Crippled my soul
My crying turned to outrage,
but by then my hands were too weak
to lift up to God or bang the door.
So I curled up in front of the big
black door of NO, crumbling,
so I could wait until God would finally let me in.
I waited so long that I starved
myself and moved toward death.
The small flicker of faith that was keeping

me alive was now nearly gone,
yet I forced myself to believe.
Then came numbness—in my fingers,
in my brain, in my heart.
There was nothing left, really.
I gave up.
It was dark.
It was night.
With no stars and no moon.
Only empty, truly empty.
I crawled away from the door and turned.
My Beloved was crawling
on the ground, just like me.
His hands bloodied, his body skin on bone,
eyes sunken, and starved,
he was somehow full of light.
He kneeled on his fragile knees,
his torso lifted, his arms wide
open in a V toward the sky.
He screamed at the top of his lungs,
"Knock, Marsha, Knock!"
Ha! He knew my name.
So I knocked at his heart.
He withstood the meager blow.
The fire inside me rapidly took over.
I was stronger than I had ever been.
My knocking turned into pounding
and pummeling his chest.
He withstood it all.
Slowly I began to reach for his wide-
open hands as I knelt, my body pressing
into His. He wrapped his fingers
around mine, and we danced.
And the dance turned into humming.
The humming became a song.
He was singing my song to me.
I closed my eyes and swayed,
His whole body swaying in support with me.
When I opened my eyes, I had drunk
what seemed like ALL of HIM,

which had merged into my body.
My beloved is mine, and I am His.
A million brightly colored doors,
all speaking my name, in voices soft,
loud, clear, muffled, called me,
"Thy will be done, Marsha, thy will be done."
I stood up. I walked to the door
of my choosing.
There was a field of high grass at the door.
I touched the doorknob, which blew
open with the wind. Swoosh. I went in.
Tall blades of grass danced with me,
touching my face.
Just like old times.
We danced together, the field and I.
He continued to sing my song for me.
Deep inside my soul was the beauty
of my heart, the wide-open door,
and my Beloved, swaying gently
with each breath I took. I was whole.
I was restored.
Amen.

Chapter 30

One day I took the necessary walk inside my kidneys.
There were dangling tendrils of frayed fabric.
Disbanded bandages, well distributed, filled the space
of each small, pea-sized organ.
The murky water was hard to navigate, but I was well used to it.
I was amazed that the waters did not cease.

I was amazed that there was any water at all.
I pushed aside tendrils only to find more, light gray and cream-colored strings,
dangling for holding on,
not quite dirty, yet I sensed they wanted something new. A new environment.
They were neutral. They were not fulfilling their function.

The tendrils were not rooted.
There was no singular life cell shooting up from the deep salty earth of my
kidneys.
There was nothing to coil around.
So they suspended themselves in hidden hope, waiting.

I walked among my tendril jungle like a warrior numbed by too much seeing.

I finally understood that every time I grasp and cling, my kidney develops
another strand of uncertainty.
I must root myself again in the horizontal flow of surrender.

It all happened so fast. Dr. T, the surgeon from Nebraska, declared that my colon and "bladder" were a mess. "You're going to need your conduit repackaged," he insisted. I thought I would be devastated. My soul knew differently. This was preparation for my kidney. I was willing. June. Yes, June would be the month.

I loved my surgeon. When I asked him if he would install a gastric tube into my belly during my bladder surgery, in order to avoid that awful tube down my throat, he reluctantly agreed.

"You have a daughter, don't you?" I asked him.

"Yes," he said embarrassedly, then quickly changed the subject. I knew the inside scoop; like requesting Ponzu sauce at a Japanese restaurant, or asking for the bank supervisor, I could get that gastric tube. Nose tube be damned!

I prepared my spirit, as usual. Prayed. Danced. Meditated. Created affirmations. Did tons of yoga. Made my visualization tape. Called friends. Got my hair and nails done the morning of admission to the hospital. Wore a fabulous dress to my hospital room. The anesthesiologist grimaced when he entered my "suite." He hesitated, then spoke with a guilty look on his face, "You know you have to drink that stuff tonight . . . you may want to wear a hospital gown."

"No thanks!" I cheerfully responded.

My dear friend arrived soon afterwards to massage my feet. Fabulous dress stayed on.

Towards evening the nurse came in with a two-liter container of liquid something or other. The boss spoke, "Okay, Marsha. Time to get to work; you need to change into a hospital gown. Here are the wipes." Surely I would not need any wipes. I mean, how bad could it be? Wouldn't toilet paper be enough? She just smiled her little smile and left me to my drinking.

After a day of fasting, plus nearly ten years of never drinking more than four cups of fluid a day, my dream night began. A dribble at first. A visit to the loo every once in a while. The constant thirst, the inklings of nausea. I was getting through. Until she brought the next two-liter bottle of liquid something or other, with the gentle instruction to "drink it all."

I eventually surrendered to the hospital gown. Each time I got up to go to the bathroom, I had to put on my prosthesis. Within an hour I was asking for not one but two portable potties. Then the rotating bedpan plan began.

Morning came, and with it the dehydration of my body, my veins retreating to the Alaskan tundra, and the IV nurse at my bedside to insert a needle for the anesthesia.

You have got to be kidding. But she wasn't. I was to be wheeled into the surgery in a few hours. Oh, how I hoped I would not have to go to the bathroom again. She found a vein and . . . I had to go to the bathroom again.

Here is how the runs work with only one leg and a hospital gown that is gaping open. I am an absolute pro. I hop to the bedpan near my bed, the one on my left side, gritting yet gently attempting to place my IV arm down on the side of the bed to help propel me to my private bathroom. Breathe in—one, two, three—plop over, landing flat on the plastic surface that by now is kind of a friend. Then, making sure the IV bag doesn't topple, and being careful so the vein doesn't blow, unabashedly get to work. I have no shame about my tiny butt. It has been well complimented in other arenas.

As they covered my head with the paper turban, I still wondered if I was going to make it to the operating room without pooing one more (or thirty more) times. My will, and the drugs, took over.

I woke up from surgery with a vibrating stomach and . . . a gastric tube! Oh, what a wonderful surgeon I had!

Other surgeons on staff came in and shook their heads. "This is highly irregular. You should have had an NG tube down your throat."

Whatever!

I put my beautiful bathrobe on and started walking around the hospital to begin my recovery. Until . . . until . . . I felt a small leak on my belly. Until my lovely, yellow, Swiss dot bathrobe began to dampen in large areas of my midsection. Until I felt burning on my left side. I told myself it was the ginger oil I was using.

Eh, it's nothing. Right?

I hadn't eaten all week, so I was hungry. First, they gave me ginger ale. I drank a cup. It immediately gushed to the bag outside my gastric tube, so I drank another and another. I drank more than I had in ten years. The nurses told me to be careful.

Yeah right, honey, when was the last time you couldn't drink for ten years?

I was doing better each day, walking miles through the hospital, getting my energy back, telling jokes with the staff. Sooner than expected, I was ready for, dun, dun, dun . . . Jell-O! I ate cherry Jell-O and guzzled down entire pitchers of ginger ale. With my gelatin cocktail in such abundance, surely ice cream was just around the corner.

The burning began. There was no gas forthcoming, therefore no solid food allowed, and therefore no early release. But I was so happy to be without the tube down my throat. So happy. So, so happy! To compensate for their need to insert tubes, they stuck another into my neck to introduce nutrition, which meant more fluid intake, which meant more difficult dialysis.

I was told to stop drinking immediately.

Noooooo! screamed the acquiescent soul.

I took a short walk the day after the feeding tube joined me. What's one more tube? I was leaking everywhere. Around my precious gastric tube, there was burning red skin. Oozing baking soda bubbles of red-infused ginger ale and molten ice chips seeped out of my belly to anywhere I might be. The nurses came to change the dressing, a few layers of gauze at first, until the geysers began.

No more drinking allowed. Period. I took to dipping my washcloth in a bowl of ice cubes for ineffective thirst quenching. My skin developed a new texture—something between desert air and volcanic ash.

I ended up flat in my bed, nurses coming every few hours to change my sheets, my gown, my dressings. Gauze, paper tape, more gauze, all layered on the left side of my belly just enough to collect the liquid. The bandages were soaked, sometimes in minutes. Boxes of textured gauze were lined up against the window, until I knew which texture of gauze worked best.

I thanked God that I was in a place where they had attentive nurses and an abundant inventory of supplies. The leaking went on for days.

Finally, an intern came to see me. "Your tube shrunk in your stomach. We just need to add some air to reanchor it."

"Will it hurt?"

"No, just pressure."

"Okay."

Hah!

All was fine, for a little while. The exhausted intern returned.

What now? I thought, but did not say. What I did say was, "Can the tube come out yet? I am starving."

"I am taking out the tube because we know you haven't eaten in ten days, but you need to lie on your right side for the entire weekend until the opening closes a bit. And you can't drink or eat. Just rest. If this doesn't work, you will be getting an NG tube."

We all knew that wasn't going to happen on my watch. Hello Ezekiel.

The "party" began. I would beat this doctor. I would win. I would show him.

First came the tingling sensation down the back of my neck. Next came the crawlies as I dared not move at all, straddled to the IV, and stuck. I would equally have to avoid calling the nurse. I might drop the call button. I lay through ten hours straight of formulaic and yet reasonably exciting *Law & Order*. A bubbly mess of soaked hospital gown was on my left by morning, slowly cooling and drying from all the burn.

I tried relaxation. Breathing in, I am breathing in; breathing out, I am . . . *get me out of here!* My skin was jumping. Was that my bone marrow itching? Hmph. How to scratch, how to scratch. No one was around that weekend.

No visitors. No family. Few phone calls. Why didn't they call? I wanted something, anything to focus on besides my little empty gastric opening. However, if I reached too far for the phone my ecosystem might be in jeopardy.

Drifting helped. Daydreaming did not help. Dialysis at least gave me something to do for four hours, as I lay there, right arm extended out, as equally bound as my left side. One small move and that would be it—treatment over, fistula clotted, surgery, more fluid.

Keep it together, Marsha, keep it together. I could, so long as there were no cramps or blood pressure drops. I preoccupied myself with the weird nephrologist who appeared for a routine visit during my dialysis treatment. Was he wearing makeup? No! Yes? I think so. He never looked at me directly.

I talked intermittently to the dialysis nurse during my treatment, trying to keep my mind alert and interested in something besides the television. When the treatment ended, I was relieved for her and for me. We had run out of niceties.

For many, many hours over the weekend, I lay there on my right side, attempting over and over to watch Peter Sellers in *The Party*. He plays a clueless but sweet man who falls for a gorgeous French beauty. Lucky for him, she seemed to like his eccentricities. My "party," except for the possibly makeup-wearing doctor, was a bit lackluster.

Sleep came and went. Mostly it went. Every moment a tiny breath to breathe, a tiny sigh of relief that I had gotten through that moment. And then the next.

If I positioned my head just right, my body wouldn't slouch into the bed. With the lack of solid food for quite some time, my minuscule frame retreated into the sheets. A nurse intern bathed me each day, changing my sheets and my gown numerous times. Small miracles. She was so thorough and conscientious. She was friends with one of my doctors, one of those doctors who seems to be comatose when dealing with patients, which was shocking because he was Irish!

My right eye pressed into the pillow. My abdominal muscles were at a standstill, so I lay and I lay and I lay. Rain came Sunday, giving me a break from the relentless sun. I wished so much that I could sleep. I wished so much that I could focus on something besides my left side. I compelled callers to stay on the line too long, trying to come up with some kind of nonsensical drama to keep the conversation interesting. There were more naps. More *Law & Order*; *60 Minutes* came on at 7:00 p.m.

I made it through the weekend. The leaking had stopped.

I watched television through the night, awaiting the approval of the Monday morning doctor to lie on my back. I was walking by Tuesday! They sent a special nurse soon afterwards to remove the nutrition tube.

By Friday I had advanced to butterscotch pudding. My hospital release came Sunday. I had a new bladder. A renewed confidence.

My body was getting ready. I drank one small cup of tea. Monday I was back at dialysis, privileged with a real pillow for my head and a bed rather than a lounge chair. Now it would only be a matter of months. A small matter that would change my days forever.

Ezekiel was paralyzed by God. Here is what he said:

"I was helpless in the hands of God.
The spirit lifted me up and took me away.
I went into bitterness and anger but the hand of God was strong upon me.
I looked and saw a hand holding out to me a scroll with writing on both sides.
It was full of sorrows."

And The Lord Spoke:
"I have made you hard and stubborn too—as tough as they are.
Son of dust, eat what I am giving you.
Eat this scroll, then go and give its messages to the people.
Go out into the valley and I will talk to you there."

Ezekiel lay on his left side for three hundred and ninety days. Ezekiel lay on his right side for forty days. He ate the bitter pill.

As Ezekiel lie there deep in his own obedience, misery, and bitterness,
his strong arm extended for all to see the potential behind his four hundred and thirty days of paralysis.
He was doing the Master's work.
He had seen the message of God in a vision of four angels,
four winds, and four wheels.
How hard could it be to endure the coming paralysis?
His sheer acceptance in doing his part on behalf of a crooked but beloved group of people carried him. Was it difficult for him to know that he had to tell the holy story whether anyone listened or not?

His head was like flinted rock, the tip of a piercing arrow, strong, unstoppable, vulnerable, laying there for anyone to see, scorn, immortalized in impunity and ridicule.
He was uncoiled.
A fire combusted in his belly, supported by a diet of whole
grains and a small amount of water.
He only spoke when God spoke.

There are few of us living the dream.

Some of us have been given the gift of uncoiling. We are always awake.
We are always uncoiling.

CHAPTER 31

The wounded heart of a weary encounterer
Sat
Waiting
For the next brick
To fall and block her path
What she really wanted
Was the next feather
To smooth itself
Along the side of her neck
So she could take a drink
Of her future
unencumbered

When I awoke from surgery . . .
When I awoke from surgery . . .
When I awoke from surgery . . .
When I awoke from surgery . . .
When I awoke from surgery . . .
When I awoke from surgery . . .
When I awoke from surgery . . .
When I awoke from surgery . . .
When I awoke from surgery . . .
When I awoke from surgery . . . I was thirsty.
I was so thirsty.

And I could not drink. I could not lift my arm.

Over and over the nurse moistened my mouth with lemon glycerin swabs.

In and out I went. From heaven to earth and back again.

"I am thirsty," I whispered. Reaching out from my scratchy throat, "Just a sip?" Would the glint of my little smile persuade her? She came back with a swab.

"You cannot drink, sweetheart."

They took out the IV when a vein blew, only to anchor it in the other arm, or leg, until it blew again. How many times? How many times?

With the new needle higher up in my arm, I could finally bend my elbow. Bend and reach. A pile of lemon glycerin swabs was left on my side cabinet, wheels locked down, drawers filled with goodies, like plastic buckets for throwing up, plastic toothbrushes, MOUTHWASH!

The swabs had plastic stick handles attached to two-inch tufts of cotton soaked in a tangy bit of moisture. If I started at the lips, rolling the lollipop along the border, beginning the descent into my inner cheeks and gums, ending finally at the tongue, I could delay the inevitable thirst. I sucked on the swab as a last resort, because then my thirst would come back full force. If only I could sleep more, then I wouldn't notice how thirsty I was.

Between the swabs and swishing with mouthwash I was satisfied for a few moments.

What would I do when the swabs or mouthwash ran out? How soon would someone come to help me?

Saline water dripped from a plastic bottle up above. Saline water to keep me hydrated, but never to quench my thirst. Washcloths made of rough terry cloth, and washed a million times in hospital-grade soap, were soaked in ice water and pressed on my face, lightly touching my tongue. Whose body fluids had they touched before? No time to think about that. Just quench my thirst. Please, quench my thirst.

Eventually came chlorine-filtered ice chips, piled high in Styrofoam cups, often accompanied by overflowing brown plastic pitchers filled with ice, rested near my bed.

"Just a few, Marsha. Give your system time," soothed the nurse.

Time. Time. TIME! So much time committed to this.

My shaky fingers dug into the cup, hoping to not knock it over. So many hospitals. So many recovery rooms. So many types of ice chips. I became a connoisseur! There were flat, flaky ice chips, elliptical ice chips with crunchy exteriors, ice chips shaped like rock candy, watery ice chips, hard-to-chew ice chips.

Sucking takes too long when you are thirsty.

Finally, a cup of ginger ale arrived. With ice chips.

"Sip it, Marsha. Give your body time to adjust."

Sip it?! Sip it!?! When would I ever be able to leave this place?

One time, in the summer of 1995, I was at the Jersey Shore, near the boardwalk, and I could no longer quench my thirst. It was my first year on dialysis. I had taken a walk on the boardwalk in ninety-degree heat. I was thirsty! Four eight-ounce cups of fluid per day was what they told me. With each cup I drank came a growing sense of guilt.

I just had to have a root beer float. The perfect vanilla cool that slid down my throat came at such a price. I could feel every swallow expand into my cells. The telltale sign was my interlocked fingers, a habit I developed soon into my dialysis journey. Could I still feel the knuckles? Would my rings fit? How much bone could I touch? By Monday I was a floating balloon—ankles and face swollen, eyes barely able to open, breath shallow and undependable—with still one more day before treatment. How was I supposed to get through an entire day without drinking? But I did. I had my tricks. A sip of water. A lemon drop. A spoonful of yogurt. A bite of apple. An-ice cold washcloth (mine, so I knew where it had been). Ice chips!

Finally, treatment came. Lots of ice chips during treatment. Until the next treatment. Should I indulge in a coffee? Yes. That was dehydrating. Or wine? Wasted fluid, and it made me puffy. Ice cream? Rarely.

"Don't forget to drink water," said the dance or yoga teacher, the massage therapist, the GP. A friend would say, "Oh, I am so thirsty. I think I'll go get some water. Want some?" Then the remembering, and the "Oh, I am so sorry. I forgot." I would watch her drink. Wonder what it was like to have a glass of water without worry.

We would joke at dialysis. "I was 'bad' this weekend."

Who would ever think that drinking more than four glasses of water in a day would be considered "bad"?

I, at least, understood, in the most minuscule way, the worry of not having enough to drink. How water simply wasn't available to me and wouldn't be. How I would just have to accept the thirst until even my desire for water disintegrated.

I thought about Jesus speaking out, "I thirst," and being so unsatisfied with the offering given.

I am not that kind of person. I did not accept the sentencing. I was not satisfied with less than. I wanted a full glass of water, even ten per day. I lived those years as if . . . as if I'd had a glass already full.

And now, finally, my glass *is* full. I haven't had an ice chip in years.

A sculptor I met in New York looked at the glossy vein slightly
hidden under the pale skin of my inner upper right bicep.
He told me my arm was beautiful,
that he wished to capture the alabaster light
and the purple blue glow of that mysterious vein.
I remembered that moment when the vascular surgeon
cut deep into the muscle fiber to draw out my fistula,
a deep vein in the arm brought to the surface for dialysis.
After losing the beauty of my left arm to GORE-TEX grafts,
lined with multiple needle marks for the first few rounds (years) of dialysis,
my right arm was my one beauty left that I did not need to hide.
Now that was being taken away, too.
While I am finished with dialysis,
therefore, no bigger 14 mm needle marks,
I am left with a bulging, bumpy ride
from inner right elbow to inner armpit.
Sometimes when I am hugged
people who do not know about the fistula tell me I am buzzing.
Good I am.
It is the constant pulse of my blood,
traveling thousands of miles every day.
I don't enjoy wearing short-sleeve shirts,
especially when I am between relationships.
Just one more scar story to tell
but I do accept the buzzing, breathing blood
that is holding so much hope for me.
Hope simply to live.
If I can live anywhere nearly as fully as the life force in that buzz
I am living the blood of Life.
A different kind of beauty maps my now-scarred right arm,
but I will forever miss its smooth surface.

CHAPTER 32

Things I Must Do After My Kidney Transplant

Leave gorgeous, alcoholic husband and get a divorce.
Write a list of dreams; create a spiderweb connecting those dreams, and do each of them.
Take up flamenco dancing.
Register my two hundred-hour yoga schools.
Dance whenever and wherever I want, every chance I get.
Finish my Shaman School and become the healer I am meant to be.
Go on match.com and learn how to date men.
Write, write, write.
Eat as many greens and drink as much water as I want.
Feel my feelings to the end and come back to inherent joy in my heart.
Receive acupuncture.
Do healing work and help change lives.
Open up.
Wear my high heels as much as possible.
Eat more chocolate.
Get a new prosthesis.
Travel to DC and create a sunset/moonset memory with my friend.
Develop new children's yoga products.
Go to a divorce support group and then be done with it.
Take up Spanish.
Paint my mermaid chair.
Make boa wreaths.
Put peacock feathers all over my house.
Paint my bedroom deep magenta.
Get a red light bulb.
Move everything out of my house that doesn't serve my spirit.
Speak up more.
Trademark more of my businesses.
Become an LLC.
Create new yoga programs.
Flirt more.

Upgrade my website.
Meet a wonderful new man.
Get stronger.
Have a voice and stand up for myself.
Learn to say no.

When you overcome a serious illness, you are expected to live every day as if it were your last, or your first! You are supposed to be grateful for every moment. Each day is an opportunity to make things even better. The future is up to you. Your life is in your hands. Only you can choose to be happy. You must think positively so your destiny will open up easily for you. Your past is just that, your past. You should live life to the limit. You better have hope for a brighter future. We're counting on you!

This is the Dream that others dream for you.

I'm a little mad about that.

Sometimes I don't want to live as if it were the very last day of my life. I don't like all that pressure to live out my impossible dreams, climb, reach, achieve, think big, be big, just in case it all comes crashing down. How long am I supposed to assuage other people's fears of their own physical demise: five years, a day, forty-one years?

What's the magic formula for overcoming multiple serious illnesses in a lifetime? Are you supposed to have five times the hope? Are you supposed to be one hundred times more grateful? Shame on you if you're not. Like that Christian woman said to me once, "How dare you complain about having cancer and losing your leg?" Peace be upon him.

How long am I supposed to live as if this were the very first day of my life? To create from scratch? To dream my world into being? To see possibility in everything? To live my life with no regrets. A day? A month? Fifty-three years?

What's the secret? Who decides what the secret is? A life coach? A pastor? A self-help guru? Your friend? You? Are you supposed to know the secret?

I'll try. Oh, how I'll try. But you know what they say. Trying is not doing.

When can I live with no beginning or ending? When can I feel that I am not missing out? When do I get to make this day count by doing absolutely nothing? When can I create absolutely no meaning in the moment? When do I get to be myself without being an inspiration to anyone? When can an experience simply be upsetting, not another lesson I must learn? When can I wear my feelings in my face without smiling because someone tells me to, especially after I just endured another round of fighting for my life?

Sometimes a girl just wants to take a nap.

Jesus had the right idea, being the alpha and the omega and all. I like the circle of eternity. There is room for a bad day in that circle.

Why not remember that, if you believe in the divine, you have no beginning and no end anyway? Why not exist in the ever now, the in-between, the endless cycle of renewal? Eternity has its perks, and first chances are one of them.

Who came up with this idea that a serious illness had to be an opportunity for a second chance at life? Why not avoid taking second chances altogether by appreciating the first chance first? Participate now.

Take a look at us chronic second-chancers if you want to understand what first chance is all about. Our dream is always the same. We would give anything to get our first chance back again.

My Soul drooped
Toward Heaven
I bowed to the heart. My heart.
I found she was scared,
Very scared.
For having to be courageous for so long,
The thought of doing it again,
Not just to stay alive and to win at overcoming.

Now the very heart of hearts. My heart
Was asking for something more.
I have found it profoundly easy, comparatively,
To get through life-threatening illnesses,
Alcoholic husband,
Severe threats to my very nature.
But this, this soul-calling awakening, this not resting,
Until she is finally heard and demonstrated throughout the world.

I just don't know if I can do it.
It is brand new.

I danced in the center today
In the center of the altar,
I held the stone of trust.
I rubbed it along my throat,
And made the pact.
I have used up a lot of energy on the rest of it,
Now I see—compassion, openness, healer, friend,
I have to be my own friend now.

I cannot abandon her when she needs me most,
I must take her out of the infertile marriage,
And place her in the fire.
I can do this.
I can find my way.
I can be with her, drooping soul and all.
I can help her take the next step.

I can show her the new possibilities
I am listening, dear one, I am listening . . .

Chapter 33

Once when the there was only Breath contemplating the moment to breathe LOVE,
everything in the universe waited to BE.
All was possibility.
So LOVE decided. "I shall breathe now."
As soon as she let out "Ah,"
the universe was born and all that lived inside it.

Back and forth the exchange went,
the deep sigh of relief in finally being born,
finally, being vibrated into form.
Every particle became a form of the Infinite breath.
There was beginning.
A leaf grew a stem and the commencement of its path to shape.
LOVE looked at all She had vibrated into form.
She felt deep unity, a love new and old,
a familiar longing finally come to pass.
She could see Herself poured out.
There was recognition.
She sang "Huuuuuu."
As she watched the wind blow, earth growl,
stars collide, the universe took from her nourishment.
She received awareness of her own emanation.
The dew rose up from the vapors.
The song was steadier now, denser, deeper. Full.
The leaf expanded to its edges, ripe and ready to be seen.
Compassion filled the heart pulse of LOVE,
for in allowing the universe to be born, there was necessary death.
The leaf was slowly eaten by another.
BREATH of LOVE paused. "Mmm." It is finished.
Only to begin again in another aspect of Herself.
Breath of LOVE knows the real truth.
She IS. Once is an illusion.
A-U-M, her eternal aspects are in constant change

as is her fixed state of BE.
If you look carefully, beyond the beyond
into the Soul of the Universe,
Breath of LOVE's long spine is central axis.
Mother Mother who am I?
You are earth
You are water
You are wind
You are fire
You are me
Love never changes.

Two days after I was sent home from my kidney transplant surgery, my very ambitious and mysterious, Clairol-induced, red-headed mother arrived with her rolling luggage. She had traipsed from New Jersey, a six-hour train ride, followed by an hour-long commuter train ride, and a twenty-minute walk in the rain to my house. It was pouring rain, almost eleven at night; she was determined, that smoking hot Irish broad.

I was so happy to see her and grateful that she'd come, even if one and a half days was all she could give. At least she wouldn't have time to set up a church singing gig, although I wasn't completely sure that wouldn't happen during this visit. Her pocketbook was stuffed full of that . . . stuff: projects she had to work on, bills she needed to pay, crossword puzzles she needed to do "to keep her mind young." I had had so many surgeries that the transplant felt like a breeze, so I did have the stamina to serve her a cup of tea with fresh-squeezed lemon and a half packet of Sweet'N Low, just the way she required it to be.

I was already beginning to feel the boiling of my blood, the tightening of my jaw as I tried to be her daughter—the kind of daughter who shouldn't expect too much. The matriarch was in my presence, and the underlying pulse in my body reminded me that if I ask for more, I won't get it, so I have to be understanding or I'll feel guilty for the asking.

There was some chatting to assuage my aching heart, but we still had to go grocery shopping the next day, and it didn't take her long to ask me what we were having for dinner. I have gotten over (mostly) the fact that my real needs could only be met haphazardly, according to the whisper of the wind. Her wind is more of a hurricane, mine more a gathering swirl of old dust. So now, three days after coming home from transplant surgery, I found myself thinking about her roasted chicken dinner, her stuffed pasta with cream sauce, her yogurt, her need to take long walks, her lengthy long-distance phone calls to all those important people, and the constant emailing to stay in touch.

She *did* drive me to the hospital, but only because I told her about fifty times that I couldn't drive for four weeks. I finally had to say, ever so humbly, "I thought you were here to help me."

It happened earlier that year, as well, with my bladder rewire surgery. My mother had come up for one and a half days then, too. A dear friend of mine offered to host "The Queen" for the two nights, but it was pretty much the same M.O., even in someone else's home. My mother arrived late that night from a very dramatic and exhausting train ride. As she walked in the door she announced that she was going to need a hot cup of tea with lemon and Sweet'N Low, and then quickly asked, "How are you doing, honey?" and "How am I getting to Mary's house?" Meanwhile, I was still on dialysis, bloated from all the fluid they'd pumped into me, in addition to the toxic feeling I carried with me after two and a half weeks in the hospital recovering from this very complicated abdominal surgery.

She had been "unable" to come see me in the hospital. What? Did she have an opera gig or something?

I never asked her to visit. She volunteered. So it came as no surprise that around 10 a.m. on the day she was leaving, she called me from my friend's house. "Hi honey, we have had such a great chat and a great breakfast. Now I am going on my one-hour walk and then you can come pick me up."

Oh. "I thought you were going to drive me to the doctor's?"

I feel so guilty and free writing this. About the years upon years of admiring her charisma, her youthfulness, her humor, her genuine kindness, her hugs, kisses, warm embraces, her confidence in me, her words of encouragement, her marabou feather nightgowns, her piano practicing, her voice scales, and her passion for all things creative.

Like a starving child with no hands to cook the meal herself. I attempted to get my sustenance from someone who placed the food in a sealed container in the freezer, promising me I would always be fed, but seldom feeding me. Every once in a while there would be such a feast, the kind that you wouldn't ever forget. I suppose that was to last me for a while until the need for sustenance was so strong perhaps she would see my wide-eyed stare at the floor.

She was (and is) loads of fun, running around the house chasing us to the music of *Peer Gynt*, spoiling us rotten with dolls, toys, cats, hamsters, trips to Paris, lunch at Tavern on the Green, all kinds of things to make us happy, satisfied, and perhaps not having to ask her for more—Will you be there for me? Will you hold me? Will you make me feel secure about this cancer or losing my leg? Will you help me decipher these friendships? Will you be my mother?

A number of years ago, I went to see an herbalist/healer in Vermont. The night before my appointment, an angel of some sort came to me in a dream and reported, "Your mother is the cause of all your health problems." Oops.

When I walked into the practitioner's office, the first thing he said was, "What is the relationship with your mother?"

"Oh," I whispered quietly. Then I told him of my dream. The ultimate guilty pleasure, revealing some truth that shouldn't be spoken.

I immediately went into all the possible reasons for the bone cancer: the environment, foods, the starvation for emotional support, diet, genetics, mystery, God (yes, as a sort of spiritual awakening from the depths of my soul), or perhaps simple neglect.

I look down at my legs and I see that the right is still here. The right one, the one that took over, had the initiative to act, but the left, well that is the receptive side, which is where the starvation went. What I could digest went to eating away my bones and, ultimately, cutting off the bone altogether.

My mother, the grande dame, the diva, often gave her grand nurturing to "those who really needed it," like troubled teens who stayed at our house for more than a year, or struggling artists and musicians, or people she'd meet on her trips. After all, we were all okay, because if we weren't, that meant acknowledging what was there: the tiniest bit of lack, the little morsel wanting to be eaten, but beyond our grasp.

My mother is a very glamorous, over-the-top woman, gorgeous beyond belief and thrilled that all of her children are as gorgeous as she is (according to her). But I suffered not from the lack of praise for my beauty; it's been my bones that have needed filling from the get-go. I am taking it in from other sources. I have found filling within me. This source is the greatest of them all. She is me and she is demanding an audience, one that will listen to the fact that her mother is a diva and that it will be okay to say so.

This is the story of the Eastern Wind, Daughter Wind.
Who asks, "When will I ever be Home?
Why do I look out across the sea to the Cliffs of Moher and my stone passageway?
Am I doing things right?"

Dance, Daughter, dance.
Arms swinging,
Feet twirling,
Spirit spinning.

That may have been where you came from, but you are here now,
So dance.

This is the Story of the Western Wind, Sister Wind.
Who asks, "When will you be comfortable in your own skin?
Why did you become a follower, where licking ice cream
has a double meaning?
And the body is another commodity, easily bought and sold?"

Dance, Sister, dance.
Move beyond the limitations,
That were never set in stone.
You know what to do.
Don't let the fear misguide you,
You've got it in you.
There was a reason the Santa Ana winds blew wide your windows.

This is the Story of the Southern Wind, Mother Wind.
The one who sings in the morning, sings all day long.
Guilt is simply sin. What are you guilty for?
Come here and let me soothe your head.
This is me. There is a huge place for you in my heart.
Dance, Daughter, dance
The one who dances in the morning dances all day long.

This is the Story of the Northern Wind, Grandmother Wind.
Live on! Pick a carrot from the field and bite deep into it.
Chew until the flavor turns to sugar. Sugar is so sweet. And you were always
my favorite.
Tea and biscuits and more tea with sugar.
Eat and dance, granddaughter.
Oh, you are so beautiful. The one who goes into the belly without pretense
Can sail across the ocean without a care in the world,
Because she is always dancing.

CHAPTER 34

Yes is not an answer
Yes is yes
My body agreeing
With what my heart
Already knows
Intuitively
Distinctly setting me apart
From my goals and aspirations
I am one with the
Unity of cells
That speak
Yes

I had received my new kidney just weeks ago. I was restless to get out of the house, so I drove to the grocery store. Both driving and shopping were not supposed to be in my vocabulary so soon after the surgery, but there I was, coming back from Stop & Shop on Route 1A, my hands and mouth coated in antibacterial lotion, thinking, thinking, thinking, for the billionth time, about whether to stay with my husband or finally leave.

When I first began to date him, eight years earlier, I would take the six-hour trip to meet him at Lake Placid, contemplating all the things that were wrong with him and us throughout the commute. I would follow that up with moments of heartfelt hope at the idea of our chance meeting, the seemingly divine setup, the abiding love. Most of the trips, though, also included *hours* of inner conversation to override the gut feelings that something just wasn't quite right.

Then *it* would happen. The rainbow. My sign of hope, of the force of love that conquers all, of God saying "yes" to my husband and me. It would all be okay. Why, then, did my palms sweat, my breath become shallow, my throat constrict? Why did terror seize me where it lived most, in my bones, and why the glaze that formed over my eyes as I continued on? Rainbows became so commonplace at the most critical moments of my inner chats about my husband that I began to expect them the moment I was about to give in to futility.

Terror is something not entirely unknown to me, nor are the physiological cues. I had simply adapted to overriding the feelings, plodding on so I could get what I wanted, which was to keep the status quo.

So it was no coincidence that at the moment when I felt myself slipping into surrender, saying, finally, that it was time to end this marriage, my precious rainbow appeared. Oh, relief. It would all be okay. We would still be together. God would see us through all this. Except that now I had a kidney. And my kidney wanted nothing to do with my marriage or my husband. So as I sat there admiring this rainbow—feeling all this hope about my husband and me and God speaking from above about how it would all work out and my husband would finally stop drinking and get his life together and we would sail off into the rainbow-infused sunset of the Maine countryside—my kidney told me to look again. The rainbow was one of the closest and the most defined rainbows I had ever witnessed. There was the answer. Two, well-defined, multicolored pillars stood at opposite ends of the rainbow. I decided that the one on the left, which was closer to me, was mine. It was much taller, brighter, and clearer than the pillar to the right. The pillar of color to the right stood tall and bright and equally independent. The arc, still softly reaching between the two pillars, was muddled, barely there, faded to the point of oblivion. It was hard to see this. I didn't want to.

When I got home there was another call from him, still not apologizing for never coming to see me in the hospital when I received this precious kidney. Instead, he told me he had made a bad decision. That's what he called it. A bad decision. Opening a restaurant not one month before, then drinking to the point of completely destroying his lifelong dream. Drinking to the point of being pulled over in his fancy truck with the stainless steel tires, the lift, and the dual exhaust. Being in jail for a week while his restaurant waited for his spectacular cooking. Being in jail while his wife, whom he adored almost as much as vodka, waited to know where he was. A bad decision? He was mucking up the rainbow, that sign from God that promised to never flood the earth again. And in his own crazy, roundabout way, he was giving me the gift of clarity. He was letting me have my kidney and my health and my hope for myself, rather than having to waste another moment on one more of his bad decisions.

So I prayed to Iris, goddess of the rainbow. I tore open decks of medicine cards, angel messages, enlightenment packs. They all said the same thing. See what's really there. Raise your consciousness. Be free. And oh, beautiful Iris, there in the wings of the rainbow cauldron, stoked my prayers with her waiting hope. Iris was the one who was willing to descend into the underworld to guide the dead to safe transition. She did it all on the arc of a rainbow.

"Eli, Eli, Lama Sabachthani?" My God, my God, why have you forsaken me?

My God, I surrender.

I have had to anchor my heart in order to stay connected to Jesus
through the struggle of leaping in and out of my body.
Over and over I have managed this.
I have managed to guard this back of my heart,
to find the root into being here, no matter what.

Oh how the space between my shoulders hurts.
My spirit has always known how to come back,
by will, by inner confidence, by spiritual design,
by total abandonment of my own agenda.

The thing is, this dance started WAY before the first round of bone cancer.
I came into this body with a deep sadness at having to leave behind

the ONE I loved.
I decided to say yes to this life, KNOWING it would be a tough one.
I decided to do it anyway.

God needed a warrior. I said I would go. I said yes.
I have always said yes, even when I was thinking no.
Yes, to the original biopsy, to the waking up from surgery.

I said yes to radiation, chemotherapy, years of living with my shorter, thinner left leg.
Yes, to bleeding in my bladder.
Yes, to the second surgery, to the amputation, to Sloan Kettering, to cystoscopies, blood tests, intravenous, bone scans, low white and red blood counts, failed bladder, a urostomy at nineteen.

Yes, to numerous prosthetic limbs, mouth sores, hairlessness through high school, blisters on my stump, pressure on my right leg, fatigue, maneuvering how I would get from one place to the other.
I said yes to high blood pressure.

Yes, to kidneys diminishing in health, yes to an ileal conduit, removal of my bladder, more tests, IVs, anesthesia, morphine. Yes, to a drink that completely cleaned out my colon. Yes, to the long scar down my middle that has been reopened four or five times. Yes, to staples in my belly, stitches deep into my skin, the permanent removal of my belly button. Yes, to blood transfusions.
Yes, to a shaved pubis and the consequent itching as my hair grew back in.
Yes, to meetings with surgeons, interns, anesthesiologists, social workers, chaplains.

Yes, to surgical hats, hospital gowns, knee-high hospital slippers, to beds that people may have died in, to bathrooms that had witnessed every type of body fluid possible.
Yes, to words that hurt, like "your kidneys are failing" and "can't I just remove your uterus? It would make the surgery so much easier." Yes, to all the catheters stuck in all those places: in my bladder, in my neck.
Yes, to a piece of bulging graft the whole length of my upper arm. Yes, to numerous surgeries to fix that piece of graft. Yes, to the failed graft, a new one in my lower right arm, a loop that was hard to the touch and painfully obvious.
Yes, to a fistula placed in my upper right arm as the lower graft failed, too.

Yes, to not taking a shower for more than four months while confined by a catheter.
Yes, to a machine to clean out my blood.
Yes, to two size 14mm needles in my arm three times per week for eleven years.

Yes, to low blood pressure, fainting, limited travel, swollen arms, puffed up body, strict and depressing diet, only four cups of fluid per day. Yes, to another ileal conduit while at the same time managing dialysis every other day. Yes, to four days of leaking acidic stomach juice that burned my skin.
Yes, to sitting in it for hours before a nurse was able to change the dressings.

Yes, to a new kidney, to another catheter down my neck, to cool leaks underneath the catheter that needed to be changed, to administration of medications through that catheter, to lots of drugs, to surgery—you guessed it, down the central line of my belly. I have said yes to it all.

The call came before I was even born. I heard that call, and I said YES.

At the gospel dance class, the teacher asked us, "Have you said yes to Jesus?" She was, as the evangelicals always are, looking straight at me. Apparently, I look like I need to be saved.

"Honey, I've said yes to Jesus so many times I need a vacation," replied my glistening eyes.

Chapter 35

I love him for the gift of keeping me from acknowledging the possible death of my own spirit through dialysis. He was doing it for me with his drinking. Someone to focus on. Someone I could judge for being ungrateful for having good health and wasting it. Someone I could pin piles of guilt on for always choosing alcohol over me. Someone whose terrible choices I could be responsible for without even trying. Someone I could agonize over, sharing intimate secrets with not-so-close friends so my suffering could be commiserated. Someone I could rescue—over and over—since my own plight was so permanent.

Someone who kept me from actively feeling and thinking about the rest of my life.
Therein lays the hope of marrying an addict.

I finally got wise. I am sorry, Jamie.

After the breakup, the walls of my home breathed again, as if they had been waiting patiently for me to return. When he left, so did the anger. There was peace.

I floundered. I had a sort of purpose with him in my life and a sort of no purpose with him gone. That night, after I found out about his lies, I took a good look at why I would pick this guy. I wrote a list naming what was wrong with him. Then I put my name in front of his shortcomings. Too salty.

That summer I visited my sister in Ohio. I made a decision. My life in Massachusetts was finished. After a divorce and a big breakup, my home needed a new tenant. I needed a new location. In September I found a realtor. By October I sold my house. By January I would be living in Ohio.

And then, I stepped on a grain of salt.

I had called my medical insurance company three separate times to be sure that I could transfer my insurance to Ohio. Each time I called I was assured that all was well.

I called one last time, right before the move, just in case.

The grain of salt had turned into a mountain.

This time there was no medical threat. There was, however, a threat to my freedom. Ohio still had a preexisting condition clause with its medical insurance policies. I wrote to an Ohio senator. I called other insurance companies. Nothing could be done until the law changed. I was not a miracle in the eyes of the insurers. I was a liability.

Freedom gone in less than a day.

Whoosh went the river. Whoosh went my body. In just a week I was without a home, without furniture, and without a destination.

The Weaver spoke.

Cape Cod kept popping into my mind. Cape Cod, where my father had married his new wife. Cape Cod, where they had a tiny condominium unoccupied in the winter.

I packed my car on January 10.

On January 11 I pulled into an ice-covered parking lot next to a car dealership and a gas station.

The next day, I put on my boots and walked along the beach.

The salty air felt good. Tears would be my new freedom.

Seeing that she had a right to cry at any moment
She began the salty journey
Of recollection

CHAPTER 36

We begin our day with the moment of decision
Should I stay underneath or expose myself to the cold
And the beauty
I choose the cold beauty
It takes time, this reckoning
For sleep
Relief from broken heart
Time
Excluding others
Away—necessary away so I can decide for myself
Unimpeded
How to fall in love with myself for the first time
It is all so new and exciting
Frightening and unnerving
Yet my nerves are getting stronger by the minute
Sweet ocean breath sunsets
Having no plan
Playing with this life as it comes
Joyful awakening to the dark and the light
Hold my hand, God.
Please hold my hand.
Amen

December 14, 2006, was the day I made the call to my soon-to-be ex. I had had enough of him, of his drinking, of our silly marriage. It was so hard to do. He seemed genuinely shocked that he had ever hurt me. Hmmm.

The only logical thing to do was to sign up for flamenco class.

I started in January 2007. Three-inch heels attached to me and my artificial leg. It took me almost an hour to get there. I only knew that it was the right thing to do.

I entered the dance space with my long, red, ruffled skirt and my black bodysuit, my hair pulled back, large hoops dangling from my ears. I felt gorgeous. The music began.

We stood diagonally, one shoulder forward, one back. Our hands arced across our body, fingers sensually moving as if through silk. Heads high. Chest up and out. And that look, eyes narrow, jaw fierce. Somewhat aggressive—well, very aggressive, and why shouldn't we be?

The Spanish singer chanted his way through countless beats. It was the off-beat, the six, that changed me forever. That and the stomping. Oh, the stomping! Heels, ball of the foot. The yeses the nos. Hands on the hips or grabbing the skirt as we spun into our own perfection. The hiding and the coming out. The dance was up to us. We only had to show what we wanted to show. The rest, well, if it was deserved.

Week after week, I went back for more stomping. Week after week, I proudly displayed my chest, my hips, my strong backbone, my presence, even my beauty. Why hide it? I moved through the dances quickly, as if my body had known them my whole life.

One day I went into Boston to take a flamenco workshop. More beautiful women, wearing ruffled skirts and cat-like glances, were spread out across the floor. The teacher taught us the dance of the "No Longer Needed Man." We stomped for a good while, swayed from side to side with that glance, reminding "him" of what he was going to miss, and then pounced, in a flash. Right hip shot up, right hand waved bye three times, tossing him (whoever he is/was)to the wind. We spun around, jumped into a plié-type squat, then grabbed our skirts between our legs, as if we had just given birth to ourselves and slithered across the floor, sweeping our skirts as we pushed the man out of our lives. A swift turn followed, and then the final blow: the lunge, the I-never-saw-it-coming split, the skirt flourishing to the left as we once and for all turned our heads to the right, finally, finally, finally getting him out of our lives. The ultimate brush-off; and it felt *so good*!

Sometimes a girl has got to do what a girl has got to do. I had been nice for far too long. I had far too much fun stomping him into the ground. Forgive me, Jesus.

There is only one painting I still need to dance.
It is the eight-by-ten-foot one hanging in the far right corner of the museum of interpretive dances.

The lady swims horizontally in the blue ocean, her thinly gauzed body revolving around itself.
Soft swirls.
Waves of freedom.
Suspended.
Deep in the ocean.

Her eyes are closed.

She has no destiny but to move with the waves.

She is every erotic creature that is afraid to dance above the sea.

I will.

Chapter 37

Things that can be taken for granted:

Getting up in the morning.
I put on my stump socks, slide into the prosthesis, yank up the sleeve.
I go to the bathroom and empty my belly with the catheter.
I walk into the kitchen, pull out the plastic bag filled with pharmaceuticals for my beautiful kidney.
Thank you so much, Jesus.

Laundry.
I open up the creaking step stool.
I stand on balanced, hip-aligned feet, a prosthetic leg that finally fits well.
I reach with confidence for the laundry basket. I have a laundry basket.
I have a washer and dryer. I have laundry.
Thank you so much, Jesus.

Wednesday, 3:00 p.m.
I work on my computer or . . .
I call a business associate or I take a walk or
I make love or I teach a yoga class or
I make faraway plans that I know I can keep.
I am not trapped inside a dialysis unit.
Thank you so much, Jesus.

A belly button
I don't recall much about her, but she used to be where the hole now is.
Hole fills up. Marsha empties. Marsha has choices now.
Thank you so much, Jesus.

A deep breath.
I almost went last year. The end of the fight. The end of the breath.
Swollen belly, swollen lungs, swollen heart. Congested to the point of death.
Please not another year of half-life.
Please not another year of double life—the one of faith pretending,

the one of no more dumping on anyone,
the one of how much more do I have to listen
to others complaining about nonissues,
the one of shhh, no envy for their ease.
Shameful girl. Where to go? Where to go.
Thank you so much, Jesus.

A car, a driveway, an electric garage door
A new kind of Thank You dangled from my keys. Thank you for nothing.

An entire spiteful day of wanting more than getting through THIS yet again.
An entire spiteful day of wanting more than "at least it's not,"
"you could be starving,"
"you could have no laundry to do."

An entire spiteful day of I don't want to be brave, courageous, hold the torch for my anxious family by being positive or not burdening anyone.

An entire spiteful day of not accepting what is, of not letting go, of not minimizing this next round of terrible suffering.

An entire spiteful day of not having to say "thank you" for a vein not popping, for my creatinine levels being relatively okay, or the postponement of an invasive medical procedure.

An entire day spent longing to shout "thank you," for something truly satisfying, and better, like well-deserved good health, financial windfalls, an engagement, a surprise bunch of red roses,
an earned trip to Paris to teach yoga.

An entire day without one more weary, drowning,
tear-soggy "I-can-find-something-good-in-this, thank you."

I wasn't planning on taking the dive that day. I had things to do, people to take care of. Just a word from a friend and the cells began to breathe. The thinking mind was left behind. The soul of my Beloved Body began to sing. There is not an unloving cell in the organs.

It came to me in the crevices of my large intestine. Somehow I had missed it before—the complete willingness, over and over, to love me back to health; to love me so much it showed me, through its stuck days and bloated afternoons, its swollen stagnant enterprise of love, absorbing, yet again, a thought, an unconscious bite, a food that it, in its infinite wisdom, was telling me not to eat.

I continued on to the liver. A garbage dump, willing, willing, willing, to take on all the trash and think nothing of it. Renewed grace for the human race and the ones who take on the hard stuff. The absorption of my suffering, my laughter, my tears, my anxiety, my bad choices, my stress, my joy.

I continued further in. Every place I went the song was the same. *Do you know how much I love you? Do you know how much I love you? Do you know how much I love you?*

Spleen, gall bladder, kidneys (all three), ovaries, uterus, small intestine, stomach, lungs, heart. The great lovers of the earth are no farther than the gurgling of your belly. I had heard this song before, in the inner heart. He had sung it to me so many times.

I understood, yet again, the nature of my living God—the lover who absorbs all suffering.

That night, I slept without dreams.

I haven't done Yoga for eight months
Just mudras and breathing
Sitting and being

I haven't done Yoga for eight months
Just receiving new body
Clearing old pathways

I haven't done Yoga for eight months
Just grieving great loss
And opening to new hope

I haven't done Yoga for eight months
Just painting and drawing
Inciting and exploring

I haven't done Yoga for eight months
Just offering words of healing
And light pouring in

I haven't done Yoga for eight months
Just preparing for a lifetime
And holding holy presence

I haven't done Yoga for eight months
Just crying from exhaustion
And seeking new ground

I haven't done Yoga for eight months
Just dancing in the center
Of all prayers and desires

I haven't done Yoga for eight months
Just lived it. Just lived it. Just lived it.
Sat Nam
(My name is Truth.)

Chapter 38

Jealousy, the emotion you are not supposed to feel.

Or is it anger? I can't remember.

God is jealous for His children.
God is zealous with love for His children.

Will you be jealous just for me for a while?
I don't want to share at the moment.

A woman who is not me finds real excitement in her life. Her dreams come true. She doesn't need to explain away her abundance. She is okay with it. She defines herself. She steps out into the adult world with a capacity to enjoy. She is able to stand her ground. She believes in herself even when she doesn't. She has responsibilities, and she meets them. She thinks well of others and herself. She supports her friends. She is invited to weddings, baby showers, birthday parties. She is not me.

I was always waiting.

I sang a song for summer camp. I created my own sparse Native American costume. She said, "Are you really going to wear that?" I liked it, so she let me. I wonder what she was doing while I sang my song. Was she even in the audience? I can't recall. I am not sure. I am never sure. She must have been there, right?

I see the movie. I feel so sorry for the kid who has to take the train back to Harlem after chemo. I cannot see that I am also left behind. I create a false independence/dependence scheme. I do whatever I want. I pursue my dreams, but I can't seem to find my way. She dangles money over me. I tell her how grateful I am all the time. Deep in the river there is anxiety about the next month and the next. Will she really show up?

I watch the pretty girl and the not-so-pretty girl get the guy. My mother has momentary insights that are right on. "It only takes one, honey." She is such a great lady. I love her.

I am afraid to call my friends. They won't want to talk to me. I shouldn't bother them. Reaching out is an unfamiliar option. I didn't know that God actually meant what He said.

I did not know how to: do laundry, open a bank account, be a committed friend, have a relationship where my real feelings were expressed.

This is one legacy I can leave behind.

My palms stayed open
Until the burning
Red of yesterday
Was no longer
An impossible
Imprint on my future
Then I prayed
Without ceasing.

CHAPTER 39

May I be happy with no constraints
May I be happy with nothing
May I be happy with all things as they are

As they are, as May I be
May I be
May I be

As if, when it appears
Differently
As if
Happiness were so

May I be happy without
Opinion
On the word—transient happiness

Questioning—happiness
Fleeting
Or always?

Was content with contentment
Was peaceful with peace
Was joyful with joy

This . . . makes me happy
That . . . makes me happy
Give me more
Always more

I think God is literally happy when she looks at me, always
Why not return the favor?

And divergence . . .

May I be hippy.
May I circle and undulate in heavy water, making it light with my whole body.
May I churn light out in all directions for everyone.

Committed. That is what I thought I wasn't when I started to study yoga in the early nineties.

Every time I stepped into that yoga class at the gym in Paris or the Peninsula Hotel in New York, I worried.

Do I take off my socks so I don't slip? Or, do I hide my leg so I won't feel so vulnerable? Do I explain my leg to my yoga classmates? Or, do I stay secretive?

I chose to be barefoot and guarded.

When my kidneys failed and I was back in New York, I was desperate to prove that I could handle dialysis and complete my PhD. Instead, when I sat down in the dialysis chair, I fell asleep almost every time I attempted to study. It could have been the material. "*Roman de la Rose*," a work of medieval French literature, isn't exactly a page turner.

When I returned to yoga in New York, I had a few more glitches to contend with than my time in France. I no longer just had a prosthetic leg to figure out, I now housed a long GORE-TEX graft on my upper left arm. This graft kept me alive. Every other day an arterial and venous needle would be stuck in that graft, pulling out dirty blood and pushing in clean blood over a four-hour period. My shoulder began to shrink on the upper left side of my body, which now leaned slightly to the right to protect my graft from being bumped.

Darling Marsha, another battle had begun. Darling girl.

It's one thing to demand extra from your adrenals when they have nice plump kidneys to rest on, not so easy when they are resting on top of kidneys that have been reduced to the size of peas. Willpower is only so strong.

I needed yoga to handle all this gobbledygook.

When I moved to Massachusetts, yoga called quickly. I took a few classes, became part of a local yoga community, and started to read everything I could about yoga. Then a pull from the heart, a few cosmic visionary dreams, and a catalogue that arrived in the mail convinced me that I would be teaching yoga soon. I found myself at an ashram in the mid-nineties, a below-knee amputee on dialysis, somehow managing a two hundred-hour immersive training with five-hour dialysis journeys at a local hospital three times per week.

Yoga coursed through every river of my being. I HAD to do this, and I didn't know why.

It wasn't easy, with the constant drops in blood pressure, the terrifying drives home from my treatment, the stops at Pizza Hut late at night, in the worst part of town, to purchase sauce-free salty cheese pizza so I wouldn't faint somewhere on a country road. I was eternally exhausted, but that did not keep me from the 6:00 a.m. yoga practices after a traumatic night at the local dialysis unit, the nosebleeds from too much heparin, the renal diet (meat and starch) at a vegetarian ashram, the limit to four eight-ounce glasses of water per day to avoid congestive heart failure, and the avoidance of all high-phosphorous, high-potassium, and high-calcium foods.

I had to do this, and I didn't know why.

Over the years, I took myriads of yoga trainings at lots of centers, carefully mapping out my dialysis schedule, my emergency route in case something happened, my necessary contacts, my food.

Something inevitably did happen.

There was that time I staggered to the ashram door (which was locked) late at night, my blood pressure so low that I knew I could faint at any moment, which meant clotted graft, a three-hour drive home to my hospital, surgery, and no more training.

There was that weekend when I had just had surgery for a new graft, forcing me to keep my right arm elevated above my shoulder, which didn't stop me from teaching a training on the chakras. Wheels were spinning, but I stayed seated, my arm resting on a chair.

There were infections, drug reactions, anaphylactic incidents, clotting, excess fluid in the lungs, bloated face, prosthetics that wouldn't fit because of extra fluid retention, catheters stuck in my neck that went directly to the heart, injuries to my residual limb, and so many other medical dramas I can't recall.

None of that stopped me from studying yoga, teaching yoga, practicing yoga.

My kidney transplant happened in 2006. Besides the divorce happening at the same time, high on my list during my first week of recovery was, "When could I teach yoga again? When could I practice yoga again?"

I started with mudras, hand gestures that work with the energy of the meridians in the body. Then came deep breathing, walking meditation, and eventually chair yoga. I was back to full-time teaching and training in four months.

Two years into my kidney transplant, I started to go into congestive heart failure, remnants of the fistula (dialysis access), which was still buzzing away in my right arm. A year's worth of worry and wonder followed. Would my kidney make it? Could I still teach yoga?

Along came mudras again! Varuna mudra to balance the water in my system. Hakini mudra to clear my mind. Gentle yoga to reduce abdominal bloating.

The doctors agreed to finally tie off the fistula. I lost ten pounds of fluid in less than three days. A week after the surgery, I was teaching a yoga training.

Yoga got me through the next big breakup, the sale of my house, medical insurance spectacles, creatinine and blood pressure frights, my shocking unscheduled move to the ice-covered roads of Cape Cod, the irritating woman I escaped in my move showing up in my yoga class on Cape Cod, elevated blood pressure, a stent surgery, another big move, loneliness, bizarre dates, and a new career helping amputees through yoga.

Who has witnessed my dedication to this yoga but me . . . and the wind?

There are moments when I doubt my commitment to yoga.

A new pair of heels or an adorable man, those I can commit to!

But yoga?

Yeah, yoga.

I am committed to yoga.

Yoga is who I am and what I do.

I am committed to yoga.

My mother is mine and I am hers
She wanders among the thorns
Until the day breaks
And the storm has passed
She watches over me

Turn, my mother
And be like a dearest friend
Or an advocate who never leaves me
How beautiful you are, my daughter
Oh, how beautiful!
All beautiful you are my daughter
There is no flaw in you

CHAPTER 40

Do not keep your tiger caged
In a dark back room
Where no one is supposed to see
That clearly you have violated
The last code of good will

You took a wild endangered animal
You hid her
She did her best to keep up her tiger ways

Now she is a trapped coyote
Mangy furred, howling.
She has nearly lost her roar

She longs to be by your side
She is dedicated to her mistress
Like a rescued dog from the gutter
But she is not yours to keep
Now you see
That the fiercest can be broken, too
Let her go!
We all know you were never meant to be alone.
Neither was she.
Let her go!
Let her go!

The tiger came back to me one day, while I was standing on the wooden balcony, my eyes parallel to pine trees, my feet adorned in shiny black heels.

That summer, he drove from Boston to my makeshift home on Cape Cod. He lived simply, after a life of hard work, drive, and discontent. Now he was following his dream, teaching science at a school in a rough part of town, doing his dandiest to survive on ten thousand dollars per year.

He never let me buy anything, which always touched me. He knew what he wanted and he got it, all without a moment of prayer. I was envious of his clarity, especially since he denied the existence of God.

In the meantime, I used every waking moment to talk to God—what, when, how, who, why?

He had such beauty with those big brown eyes, dark brown skin, and black hair.

Such sweetness, such compassion, such loveliness exploded on his face.

His subtle Indian nature, refined yet wild, sensual yet tame, compelled me.

A good boy. He was a good boy.

He was my first summer romance. Ever.

Every moment with him was precious.

And insightful.

This was the summer of the job at the lingerie store, the cute outfits, and the daily run to buy the best decaf soy cappuccino I've ever had.

This was the summer of sticky sand in toes and hair, secret moments I will never repeat, and music.

This was the summer of drinks in the middle of the day, sexy encounters at surprising locations, and extra dessert, often.

He called himself a tiger.

But I knew who the real tiger was.

That summer I let her out . . . a little bit.